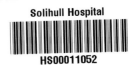

Fighting Fatigue

Fighting Fatigue

a practical guide to managing the symptoms of CFS/ME

Edited by
Sue Pemberton
and
Catherine Berry

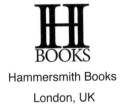

Hammersmith Books
London, UK

First published in 2009 by Hammersmith Press Limited
Published by Hammersmith Books Limited since 2015 in print and ebook formats
4/4A Bloomsbury Square, London WC1A 2RP, UK
Reprinted in 2010, 2011, 2012, 2014, (and by Hammersmith Books) 2016, 2017
www.hammersmithbooks.co.uk

Whilst the advice and information in this book are believed to be true and accurate at the date of going to press, neither the authors nor the publisher can accept any legal responsibility or liability for any errors or omissions that may have been made. In particular (but without limiting the generality of the preceding disclaimer) every effort has been made to check practical instructions; however, it is still possible that errors may have been missed. Furthermore, treatment schedules are necessarily particular to the individual and are constantly being revised and new side effects recognized. For these reasons readers are strongly urged to consult a health professional with regard to specific treatment.

British Library Cataloguing in Publication Data: A CIP record of this book is available from the British Library.

Print ISBN 978-1-905140-28-2
Ebook ISBN 978-1-78161-022-0

Commissioning editor: Georgina Bentliff
Designed by Julie Bennett
Typeset by Julie Bennett
Production by Helen Whitehorn, Pathmedia
Printed and bound by TJ International Ltd
Illustrations by Peter Hudspith
Front cover photograph by Angela Bann

Contents

Contents

Contents

Chapter Seven Memory and concentration 150
By Sue Stanley and Lisa Hinds

Chapter Eight Dealing with others 165
By Ian Portlock

Contents

Contents

Acknowledgements

This book is the result of our work over the past 18 years; if I acknowledged every person individually who has helped us on this journey there would be no room left for the contents. So, instead I would like to thank every professional who has been part of the Leeds & West Yorkshire CFS/ME Service over that time, for your commitment to and enthusiasm for helping people with this difficult condition. All your ideas and contributions have helped us to develop the strategies we use within therapy and that we are sharing with others through this book. I would particularly like to thank the current team, both those listed as authors and those behind the scenes, who have worked so hard to turn the material that we use in our clinical practice into a book that everyone can read. Also, thank you to Dr Hiroko Akagi and Dr Diane Cox for their additional contributions.

I would like to acknowledge the support that the service has received from the Leeds Partnership NHS Foundation Trust, which has ensured that we have survived and grown through the years. I would like to thank Catherine for inspiring us to share our knowledge and then working so hard to make this a reality. Also, thank you to Georgina Bentliff and the team at Hammersmith Press for believing in our idea.

Most importantly I would like to thank the thousands of patients who have given us knowledge and understanding of their experiences. You help us to continue learning about the things that do and do not support your recovery. Many of you have given your time and energy to help with the development of the service, contributing to the clinical booklets that form the basis of this book. I would particularly like to thank those of you who have given your stories in the hope that they will help others on the same journey. Finally, to my family, thank you for everything.

SP, 2009

I first experienced the symptoms of CFS/ME in 1998. For seven years I looked around for answers as to why I felt so poorly and for advice on how to feel better. I heard about the Leeds & West Yorkshire CFS/ME Service through a friend of mine. I attended the service throughout 2006 and experienced significant benefits to my health as a result of applying their management strategies. At the end of 2006 I talked to Sue about putting the information into a book so anyone with CFS/ME who cannot access the service can still benefit from their approach.

I know the encouragement from others supported my recovery. It is our intention that the stories of people who have benefited from the strategies in this book will be a source of encouragement. Thank you to Heather Mundill, Georgina Hambling, Jill Clark, Lisa Kavanagh, Lee Crust, David Incoll, Sue Johnson and others who have been willing to share their experiences as a source of support for others.

Thank you to Simon, who has stood by me. In difficult times we continue to love each other and I am grateful for all you have given. Thank you to Dad, who always believed in me. Thank you to Mum, who is the most patient person I know. Thank you to Richard, a rock in my life. Thank you to Victoria, who is more than she realises she is. Thank you to Claire who was a light when the darkness of CFS/ME was in my life.

Thank you to Sue, who understands. Thank you to Sue's team. Thank you to Angela Bann for creating the photograph for the cover of this book. Thank you to Georgina and Hammersmith Press for supporting this book.

CB, 2009

About the Authors and Editors

Catherine Berry

Catherine has suffered from CFS/ME for the past nine years. Over that time she has followed many different treatment options in the hope that they would improve her health. She researched the condition on the internet and read several books that claimed to improve the health of sufferers. Nothing seemed to offer practical solutions to the problem. She attended the Leeds & West Yorkshire CFS/ME Service in 2006 and since completing the programme her health has significantly improved. She is keen for the information about the programme to be available to all those sufferers who are not able to attend the service personally.

Penny Forsyth

Penny is a Chartered Physiotherapist with eight years' experience of working with people with CFS/ME in outpatient, inpatient and community settings. She works with several multidisciplinary teams in Leeds delivering advice and education to people suffering from the condition as well as treating individuals.

Lisa Hinds

Lisa qualified from York St John University as an occupational therapist in 2004. She then worked across a variety of health care settings gaining experience with people who had acute and chronic mental health problems before moving to her current post at the Leeds & West Yorkshire CFS/ME Service in 2006, where she works as a senior occupational therapist. At present, she is studying health psychology at postgraduate level and has a particular interest in how personality and individual differences affect adaptation to chronic illness. As part of her studies she is keen to learn how health conditions, such as CFS/ME, affect cognitive functioning.

Katie Lorentz

Katie is a qualified occupational therapist with nine years' experience working in the NHS, the last four of which have been with the Leeds & West Yorkshire CFS/ME Service. Throughout this time Katie has worked with people with a variety of health problems and become aware of the additional difficulties and unpleasant symptoms that stress can create. Katie has worked with people on understanding the stress that they experience and the impact that this has on their lives and ability to cope with their ill health. This understanding then leads to the opportunity to develop strategies for managing the condition differently.

Suzanne Moore

Suzanne works as a clinical nurse specialist in cognitive behavioural therapy at the Leeds & West Yorkshire CFS/ME Service. After qualifying as a mental health nurse in 1985, Suzanne trained as a cognitive behavioural therapist in 1995. She has since developed clinical expertise in delivering cognitive behavioural therapy (CBT) within the specialty of liaison psychiatry, having a special interest in chronic fatigue. Suzanne provides CBT to individuals and has also delivered mindfulness based cognitive therapy to groups within the service. She is experienced at delivering CBT training and supervision to a range of professional groups.

Sue Pemberton

Sue is a qualified occupational therapist who was involved in setting up the Leeds based CFS service in 1990, one of the first NHS clinics specifically for the condition. She wrote the original therapy programme and has worked clinically with the service throughout its history. Sue is currently the Clinical Champion for the condition for the North, East and West Yorkshire area and contributes to collaborative work nationally in this field. She is the only consultant occupational therapist working in CFS/ME in the country, speaking regularly at national conferences on the condition and contributing to the national training of health professionals.

Louise Penny

Louise has worked as a Registered Mental Health Nurse for the past 24 years and transferred her skills to work within the CFS/ME Service four years ago. Louise has always recognised the important role family members and friends undertake when caring. During her nursing career she has worked closely with patients, families and carers both in the hospital setting and within their homes; this work focuses on supporting carers, educating them in managing illness and helping them to recognise their own needs as carers.

Ian Portlock

Ian is a specialist occupational therapist who has been part of the Leeds & West Yorkshire CFS/ME service for four years. He has worked with many people with CFS/ME in that time, both in individual settings and within groups. Improving the areas of sleep and dealing with others has been an important part of managing CFS/ME for many of the people Ian has worked with. The experience and knowledge of the patients and clinicians Ian has spent time with has been vital in developing these chapters.

Clare Redmond

Clare is a Specialist Registrar in psychiatry, currently working in the Yorkshire region. She obtained her medical degree from Leeds University in 1998 and went on to specialise in psychiatry, becoming a member of the Royal College of Psychiatrists in 2004. From 2006 to 2008 Clare worked with the Leeds & West Yorkshire CFS/ME Service and developed an interest in the way that depression and anxiety can affect those with CFS/ME.

Sue Stanley

Sue graduated from York St John University in 2000. She is a qualified occupational therapist who has worked in ward and community based settings. She developed an interest in how cognitive impairment impacts on occupational performance when working with older age adults. In 2004 she moved to her current post at the Leeds & West Yorkshire CFS/ME service, where she works as a senior occupational therapist

Introduction

Many of you who pick up this book will be feeling alone and confused. You may have gone from being fit and healthy to now struggling to get out of bed. It may seem that no one can tell you why. Do you ask yourself why the life you had before you became ill appears to be suddenly falling apart? Despite all your efforts to keep going, your body is letting you down. You may be battling to find answers. 'Maybe I still have the flu?' 'Maybe I need more vitamins?' 'Maybe I need a holiday?' It can seem that nothing you try makes any difference. It can feel worse if no one around you understands how you are feeling. However, many people do know exactly how you are feeling and have been through that daily battle. They also know that you can fight fatigue and win. However, you need to fight it differently. This book includes their stories so that they can help you along your road to recovery.

Chronic fatigue syndrome/myalgic encephalomyelitis (CFS/ME) is a condition that affects approximately 180,000 people in the UK. It is characterised by persistent and unusual tiredness, which is made worse by any physical and/or mental activity. Alongside this people also commonly experience a range of other symptoms, including muscle pain, headaches, sleep disturbance, loss of concentration and memory, sore throats and swollen glands (NICE, 2007). However, people describe many different changes and symptoms that can happen alongside the fatigue, such as digestive problems, sensitivity to light and noise, poor temperature control, and many, many more.

It does affect people differently, from mild cases, where the person struggles to continue working, to the most severe, where the sufferer cannot get out of bed. Although CFS/ME is recognised by the World Health Organisation as a neurological condition, there are still many aspects of this disabling problem that we do not understand. There is a growing awareness of the condition, supported by the recent publication of NICE guidelines (2007) on its diagnosis and management, but specialist healthcare is still scarce and many people have to use their own resources to fight it.

Please remember that *Fighting Fatigue* is not a substitute for obtaining a formal diagnosis from your GP or other qualified health professional. If you are experiencing symptoms of fatigue it is essential that you rule out other possible causes before embarking on the self-help strategies described here. The book does not cover issues about the nature of the condition, how the diagnosis is made or possible causes.

Fighting Fatigue provides guidance to people who have been given a diagnosis, their carers, and professionals, on self-help strategies for managing the condition. The book is based upon booklets, which are a key part of the therapy process, developed over the last 18 years by the multidisciplinary team at the Leeds & West Yorkshire CFS/ME Service. The clinical information is enhanced by real-life stories of people who have attended the clinic and used the strategies themselves. These stories will help to encourage and support you if you are suffering from CFS/ME, as they are written by people who have shared your experience.

If you have been given a diagnosis of CFS/ME, this book is designed to be a useful tool in your recovery. It gives straightforward and specific advice on managing different aspects of everyday life that can affect energy. Each of the 11 chapters focuses on a different area and gives expert advice on that topic accompanied by real-life stories from people who have used this. The book asks you to put the advice into practice and helps you to work through the programme. It has been written by people who understand the way fatigue affects concentration. Therefore, it is broken into easy to follow steps so that you can work through it at your own pace. Each chapter begins with a summary sheet that lists all the sections within the chapter. You can tick off the sections you have read and the tasks that you have completed, recording which you have found helpful. You may wish to photocopy some of the worksheets before you write on them, so that you can use them more than once. Copies of the key ones are also available on the publisher's website (www.hammersmithpress.co.uk).

We advise you to work through *Fighting Fatigue* slowly and think about each idea. Although this may seem like a difficult task if you look at the book as a whole, please remember it has been written by people who understand your condition. It is designed to be worked through in small steps and has a star system to guide you, with ✳ to mark the end of each of the sections. When you reach a star it is a good idea to stop at that point. Take time to think about what you have read. You may find it useful to come back to the book at another time and re-read a section, to make sure you have understood each part before you move on. The key strategies for managing CFS/ME are covered in the first chapter. After that you do not need to read the chapters in order, but can focus first on the areas that are most relevant to you.

If you are struggling due to problems with mental fatigue and tend to lose concentration after reading for a while, the following techniques may help you to read this book.

Think about how much you can generally read before your fatigue level starts to increase. For some people it is one page (or just a paragraph); for others it is 10 pages or more.

Stop reading when you have read the number of pages you can manage without increasing your mental fatigue. Mark the point you have reached.

Put the book down at this point and do something else or rest for a significant period of time.

Come back to the book. Again, only read the number of pages or paragraphs you can read without increasing your mental fatigue at one time.

We hope that you find *Fighting Fatigue* a useful tool within your recovery. Remember your energy is precious; before you had a wealth of it and could spend it as you wished; now you have to look after the little that remains. You will need to spend it wisely, helping it to grow again and also learning that sometimes getting something you really want will be worth it!

The Editors, 2009

Reference

NICE (National Institute for Clinical Effectiveness) (2007) *Chronic Fatigue Syndrome/Myalgic Encephalomyelitis (or Encephalopathy): diagnosis and management of CFS/ME in adults and children*. London: NICE

Chapter One

Managing your daily activity and energy

Sue Pemberton

Introduction

Thinking about and planning your daily activities are key concepts in the management of fatigue. You may have already cut back on the activities you are doing everyday but find that you are still experiencing high levels of fatigue and pain. You may be doubtful that working on managing your daily activities will make any difference to how you feel. Your daily physical, mental and social activities, however, do directly affect the symptoms you experience. To manage your energy effectively you will need to examine the components of your everyday life and break them down into achievable steps. Actively managing your energy and activity each day will help you to stabilise and gradually increase your energy levels. This will give you back a sense of control over your condition.

This chapter focuses on how to think about the activities that you do every day and then how gradually to increase your level of activity as part of your recovery from CFS/ME. Within the real world, grading or pacing what we do is very difficult. There are lots of things within our lives that we cannot predict, or feel we cannot control. You may come across problems that you find difficult to solve. This chapter is designed to help you to look in more detail at how to overcome any obstacles. On the next page is a list of the sections contained within this chapter. The columns on the right allow you to tick off the sections you have read. You can note which techniques you have tried and record if you have found them helpful. For most people, it is a combination of factors which can help to improve their activity levels.

Summary Sheet

Topic	Read	Comments
Introduction		
Your human battery		
How am I spending my energy?		
Why is doing things not as easy as it seems?		
Making activity work for you		
The microscope approach – setting your baseline		
Using an activity diary		
Reviewing your activity diaries		
The helicopter view – seeing the bigger picture		
Making changes – the principles of how to grade your activity		
Breaking down activity – ways to grade		
The dangers of the 'starter-finisher'		

Setting your stopping point		
Combining activities		
Making the grade		
What if it goes wrong?		

Why is managing your activity important in relation to your fatigue?

There are many aspects of the cause and biological processes of CFS/ME that are currently unknown. However, a common feature that people who have the condition describe is that they have a limited supply of energy to serve the needs of their body. This is a constant problem, but the level of fatigue can also vary and is worsened by increased levels of physical, mental and emotional exertion or activity.

Every task you undertake, from getting out of bed each morning to undressing for bed at night, requires energy. It is a simple question of 'supply and demand'. If your energy supply is low or disrupted and activity levels are high, your body cannot meet the demands of your life. In CFS/ME the severe drop in energy capacity means that even minimal activity can lead to prolonged periods of fatigue.

The following analogy may help you to understand the importance of how you manage the energy that you do have and its impact on your health. Often people use the comparison with having a 'battery' that has developed a fault, when they are trying to explain to others how they feel when they have fatigue. Also, they use this to explain why they do not just recover when they rest or sleep, like other people do when they are 'tired'. In CFS/ME we do not understand what causes the fault in the battery yet, but how you use the energy left in the battery can affect the symptoms of your condition.

Your human battery

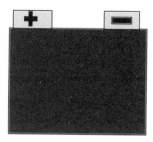

People often associate the concept of energy with 'batteries' and will describe that having fatigue makes them feel like they have a 'flat battery'. However, in the human body this 'battery' is not in one organ nor does it involve just one biological process. Many of the body's systems have a role to play in producing or mobilising energy – for example, your respiratory and circulatory system get oxygen into and around your body providing energy, your digestive system releases energy from food, your hormones can regulate your energy supplies and your nervous system instructs your body parts to function and use energy.

There are many health conditions which can cause problems with fatigue. Sometimes these are due to a specific problem occurring in the body. For example, when someone is anaemic their red blood cells do not have enough iron to help store and carry oxygen around the body. This makes the person feel fatigued. In this case there is a specific problem stopping the body producing the energy needed. When the problem is corrected, by having more iron, the fatigue goes away. With CFS/ME, all of your body's systems seem to be affected. People describe a wide range of symptoms, in addition to the primary problem of fatigue, with symptoms varying from day to day. With CFS/ME we cannot find one specific part of the body that if we mend then the problem is fixed. In this way it can be compared to there being a 'system' problem with the way your 'battery' is working. So we are going to focus on improving the overall functioning of your 'battery'. We want to help energy to be produced and watch how much energy is being used.

People with CFS/ME often describe having fluctuating levels of energy. Even on the 'good' days their energy levels are still significantly lower than before having the condition. This can be illustrated on the battery by a low level of charge, showing there is only a little left.

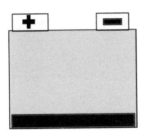

Many people who get CFS/ME describe having had highly active lifestyles before they became ill. They are often people who like to be 'doing' and find it difficult to switch off and relax. They also have a tendency to prioritise the needs of others. Therefore, they would spend their energy in the past on helping other people, such as family or work colleagues. Usually they like to 'get the job done' and to complete work to a good standard. This means they find it difficult to do only part of a task, or even to attempt activities, if they know they are not able to give it their best.

So, despite having low energy levels due to CFS/ME, on the days that they feel they have some energy, however small, they may try to do as much as they can while the energy is there and push past their limits. Also they may feel guilty when they think that they are 'doing nothing', especially if the people around them are busy. We are going to look more at what *you* are doing on page 17.

How your energy is used up

The natural pattern of someone with CFS/ME is to be as active as possible when the energy is there, which in turn 'flattens the battery'. When the battery has been flattened, then there is no choice but to rest or stop activity in order to 'recharge'. This pattern is often called a 'boom and bust' pattern of activity.

Alternatively, some people try to avoid flattening the battery by staying within very small activity levels. This helps to avoid the dead battery situation but means they can feel stuck at this level and may worry about how to do more, in case the battery starts to go flat again.

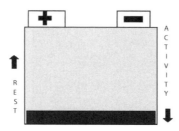

How to ration your energy

Managing your activity can ration energy, by trying to use it to best effect. The intention is to avoid flattening the battery and allow opportunities to build energy levels over time. This is done by using smaller amounts of energy at any one time and spreading the total energy used out over longer periods. This may mean prioritising the most important tasks or finding alternative ways to do things, which can conserve or reduce the energy required. So if you do smaller amounts of activity, so that you do not use up all the supply in your battery, this leaves some energy that your body can build on or use for other activities.

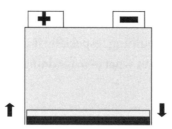

How to increase your energy supply

Managing your activity also involves looking at ways to generate energy by recharging your battery, as well as thinking about how you spend your energy.

For example, it is important to explore what happens in between periods of activity, in addition to what you are doing. People often believe that sitting or lying down is *rest*. It is important to understand the difference between stopping physical movement and actually *relaxing*. Relaxation strategies can be used to improve the quality of 'rest', which will help the production of energy. People with CFS/ME often say that when they are sitting down *resting* their minds are still very active. They are thinking about the things they should be doing. Learning how to relax both your mind and body can help with recharging your battery. Further advice on relaxation is available in Chapter 5. There are also other ways to improve your supply of energy, which we will look at later in this chapter.

How to jump start your battery

We also have back-up emergency supplies of energy. We use these when we are in a crisis or when we really need to push ourselves to do something important to us. In these situations we can use our body's emergency response system, which is described in more detail in the chapter on Stress and Relaxation, to produce short-term supplies of energy. Some people refer to this as 'running on adrenalin'.

This may help you to get through a particular situation but will increase your fatigue levels afterwards, as your body recovers from this. For example, if there was suddenly a crisis you would have a sudden boost of energy to help you to deal with this. Once the situation was less urgent and the adrenalin levels had reduced, you might then begin to experience increased fatigue.

Sometimes using this additional boost can be helpful, as it may enable you to do something you really want to do and so feel better in yourself. However, you know you will need to increase your rest afterwards. If you were doing this all of the time it would not help your recovery. This is just like eating some chocolate cake when you are dieting - you can get away with it sometimes, but not all of the time!

Useful questions to ask yourself:
- Do I flatten my battery or am I stopping before this happens?
- Could I use my energy differently?
- When I rest do I really relax or do I just sit/lie down?

How are you spending your energy?

Before we start to look at how to change your daily activities to help your fatigue, you first need to understand more about the things that you do each day. Usually in life we do things without thinking about them first - our everyday life becomes automatic. The first lesson with fatigue is that you have to **think before you do**. This can be very difficult when you are so used to just getting on with life. The first problem is that most of us do not realise the number of complicated processes and factors which all have to work together to enable us to do even a simple task, such as writing a letter.

Although you do not need to understand all the changes that occur in your body to allow it to move and function, it is important for you to be aware of the variety of factors that can influence your ability to perform a given task. People who have CFS/ME often say they have 'done nothing all day' because they are comparing themselves with their previous lifestyles. They do not think about the way small, everyday jobs can affect their fatigue.

Also, you may be unable to identify anything in your routine that has led to an increase in your fatigue because you are focusing on physical activities alone. People often forget that energy is needed for all types of activity, including emotional, mental and social tasks. Therefore, the first step is to become more aware of your everyday life and the energy that is needed for all the things you do.

The following task asks you to start to think about the energy requirements of everyday activities.

Task

Using the worksheet on the next page, write a list of all the activities that you can think of, whether you are currently able to do them or not. Think as broadly as you can. Then, work through your list, and tick whether you think each activity is **high, medium, or low**, in relation to its energy requirements for you. This can be either mental or physical energy.

You can choose to do this task based on how you currently view each activity or how you viewed it before you had fatigue. If you would currently rate everything as high, then it would be more helpful to consider how you would have judged them before you became ill.

You can assign an activity to more than one category if you feel that other circumstances may determine how much energy the activity would require. For example, if you felt that walking could be high, medium or low, depending on whether you were walking around the house, going to the shops, or going on a strenuous walk, then you might tick all three.

Adapted from Cox DL (2000) *Chronic Fatigue Syndrome and Occupational Therapy*. London: Whurr

For example:

Activity	High	Medium	Low
Getting dressed		✓	
Washing up	✓	✓	
Phoning a friend		✓	✓
Paying bills / organising money	✓	✓	
Watching TV			✓
Driving the car	✓		

Activity	High	Medium	Low

Adapted from Cox DL (2000) *Chronic Fatigue Syndrome and Occupational Therapy.* London: Whurr

The list you have written will not cover all the things you do in life but it will help you to start to think about how different tasks need different levels of energy. This will not be the same for everyone. Some people may think that using a computer is a low energy activity. This may be because they are used to doing this, or they may only be doing things on the computer that do not require much concentration, or they may just enjoy it. However, someone else may find this a high energy activity. This may be because they find concentrating more difficult, or are not used to it, or do not like using computers. Think about the things that have influenced your decisions about whether to tick high, medium or low for each activity.

Useful questions to ask yourself:
- Are there any aspects of the task itself that make it harder, such as standing for a long time?
- Did your experience of the activity before having CFS/ME make any difference?
- Do you generally find particular types of tasks harder, such as physical or mental tasks?
- Did it *depend* on lots of other things, such as:
     - where you were doing it?
     - whether other people were involved?
     - when you were doing it?
     - whether it was a good day or a bad day?
- Did whether you like or enjoy the task make any difference?
- Was it harder if emotions were involved, such as stress or conflict, or when doing it to meet other peoples' expectations?

✳ It is only by questioning yourself that you will start to increase your awareness of the complicated nature of apparently simple things. This is why when you try to do things differently you can find there are no magic formulas or simple answers. You need to learn how to think about activity and how it affects you and your fatigue. This will be different to how it can affect someone else with the same condition.

In the remainder of this section we will look at how to think about activity in more depth and some of the ways to change how you live your daily life. You will need to experiment with activity to find the right balance for you.

Why is doing things not as easy as it seems?

When you are fit and healthy, doing everyday things seems easy. Most people with CFS/ME feel frustrated at not being able to do even simple tasks, such as washing their hair or reading the paper. It is only when you lose your energy that you really start to appreciate how much energy such seemingly basic jobs take. If you stop to think about how many different things are involved in doing an activity, you can begin to realise how complicated daily life really is.

For you to complete a simple job, such as making a cup of tea, lots of different processes have to work together. Below is just an example of a few of these things.

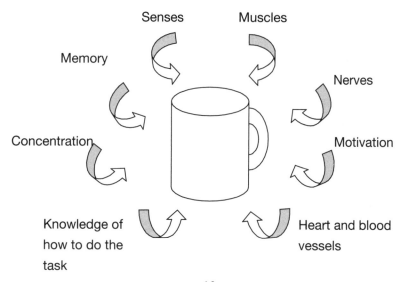

Senses   Muscles

Memory

Nerves

Concentration

Motivation

Knowledge of how to do the task

Heart and blood vessels

- **Biomechanical**

  This refers to how your body moves. In simple terms the brain sends signals through the nerves to the muscles, which move the joints. In order to make one movement, like lifting your arm with the kettle, a complicated pattern of different muscles tensing, whilst others relax, needs to occur in the right order to make this happen. Feedback needs to go back to the brain through the senses and nerves to allow the brain to make adjustments to the movement.

- **Physiological**

  Your body needs to adjust its internal systems in response to your activity. For example, your heart rate may increase, the amount of oxygen in your blood may change, chemicals may be released or other responses may happen.

- **Sensory**

  Your brain gets a constant stream of information about what is happening both inside and outside of your body, through your senses. Your senses, such as vision, hearing, touch, smell and taste, help you to adjust your actions and keep you safe. For example, making sure you are pouring the hot water into the cup. Your internal sensors, such as those for identifying pain or pressure, alert your brain to any danger or change. You also have other sensors that help you to know where you are in relation to space and gravity, such as knowing the position of your joints and keeping your balance.

- **Cognitive processing**

  Your brain interprets the information it receives and uses your memory, perception and decision-making centres to co-ordinate movement and determine your actions. Your brain needs to sequence a series of different actions in order to complete the task based on what it has learnt from the past.

- **Emotional**

  Your emotional state can affect your performance of an activity. For example, if you are upset or anxious you might shake and spill your drink, or you may not want to do the activity at all.

As well as your internal processes there are also external factors that can affect how you do a task.

- **Social**
  The context in which the activity occurs can change how we perform it. For example, it may be easier to make a cup of tea for yourself than in front of a group of people.
- **Environmental**
  Where you do the activity can also make a difference. For example, whether it is too hot or cold, do you have to stand or sit down, is there enough light to see or is it too bright?

In addition, there are other factors around your individual relationship to that activity which can make a difference, for example:

- **History** – what is your past experience and skill in the activity?
- **Self-esteem** – what are your thoughts and expectations of yourself in relation to the task?
- **Reward and purpose** – what is its meaning and purpose for you?
- **Roles and relationships** – how does it define the person you are and how you relate to others?
- **Financial** – are there any financial consequences of the activity?
- **Spiritual** – how does the activity itself or the way you carry it out relate to your belief system?
- **Cultural** – what is the meaning of the activity within your social group?

All of these things are therefore involved in what you do and how you do it. Why you are having difficulty with an activity could relate to one or many of these factors. As you start to look at patterns of activity and using energy more effectively, remember it can take time to find the right solutions - doing even simple things can be so complicated!

Making activity work for you

Once you start to understand all the different things in your everyday life that require your energy, you can start to think about how you could make changes to maximise the energy that you have. The way you did an activity in the past may have worked for you then, but does it work for you now? Could you do some tasks differently to reduce the amount of energy it takes to do them? For example, sitting to do a task rather than standing, or getting other people involved.

No two individuals are the same. This seems like an obvious statement but it is amazing how many of us compare ourselves with others, or with our own past achievements, and then feel frustrated. The problem is that many people who have CFS/ME previously were highly active and were always doing something! At the moment you may be feeling that you 'can't do anything', because you are comparing yourself with how you were in the past. The starting point for improvement is first to look at the here and now. If you do not have a clear picture of what is happening now, how do you know what to change? How will you know if you have changed it?

In the next stage of the process you can start to look at your daily life and where your energy is going each day. Find areas that you could adapt or change. We are going to look at whether you can break down the activities you are doing to make them more manageable. This is often known as *pacing*. Once you have achieved this you can then think about how you can start to make small, manageable increases to your activity levels. This is often known as *grading*.

People have different ways of looking at things. We have included two different approaches to understanding your patterns of activity. The first is taking the *microscope* view. This involves looking in detail at each day, each activity that you do and how this affects your fatigue. The second takes a *helicopter* view. This looks at the bigger picture of the different demands on your energy supply. These two approaches should begin to help you to clarify what is happening in your life.

The microscope approach - setting your baseline

If you think of this in terms of a journey, the baseline is the departure point, or it is like building the foundations for a house. The challenge is finding the right place to start. Your fatigue levels will vary; so on some days you may be able to do more than others. This is the typical 'boom and bust' pattern associated with CFS/ME, illustrated by the dotted line in the next diagram. At times, you may feel that you have a little bit more energy and so do things while you can. This leads to periods of increased fatigue, meaning you then have to rest.

With a baseline, you are trying to find a level of activity that you can manage that does not cause excessive levels of fatigue. Your fatigue level will still fluctuate, as illustrated by the central line, but by avoiding over activity or excessive rest it stays in a more stable range. However, what is 'over activity' or 'excessive rest' will be different for each person, so finding your baseline is a difficult process and you have to find what works for you.

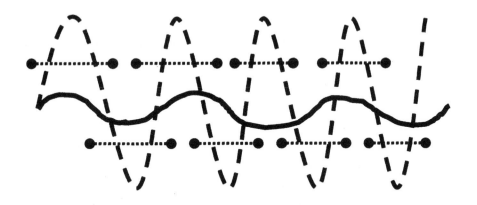

- - - - Energy fluctuation in a boom and bust pattern
———— Energy fluctuation at baseline
• • • • • • • Setting maximum and minimum activity levels

Many people do not know where to start in finding their baseline. Some people do what they can manage on a good day, everyday, and this does not work. Others may follow what they feel their body is telling them to do, which can help to stabilise the symptoms but they do not seem to be making progress. To know where to start you need to know what you are currently doing. The next section focuses on how really to understand where your energy is going.

Using an activity diary

An activity diary is a record of how your time has been spent during the day. The important factors to know are what you did, for how long, and what happened to your fatigue or other prominent symptoms.

Warning – everyone can struggle to remember all the things they have done in a day, so when you add in the memory problems with CFS/ME, if you do not write down what you have done you are likely to misjudge it. It will take energy to keep a diary, but if you can manage this, it is likely to save you energy overall.

The way that you get this information can be as simple or complex as you make it. Some people prefer to keep a detailed daily diary, and so require plenty of space to add descriptions. Others find this too time consuming and like to use general terms.

Use whichever approach suits you and to help you, a standard format has been included in this book. It is useful to see the week as a whole because your fatigue can often be delayed. Therefore, it is important to be able to identify the things that you did before your fatigue increased.

Task

Use an activity diary to record your daily life over the period of a week. A version of a diary has been included here.

• Use arrows to show how long each activity lasted or write the time it took next to each one.
• Make sure that you record rest periods through the day and the times you get up and go to bed.
• Use the fatigue scale to rate your fatigue as you go through the day. Think of 10 as the worst you have felt since experiencing fatigue and 1 as no fatigue. As you record each activity in your diary think about how far along the scale between 1 and 10 you are at that time.

Note: This is not a scientific measure and cannot be used to compare your fatigue to that of others. However, it will help you, over time, to assess if your fatigue levels are reducing.

For example:

Times	Monday	Tuesday
7.00 – 8.00	Asleep	Asleep
8.00 – 9.00	Woke 8.30 am; lay in bed 30 mins **8**	Woke, did stretching in bed **7**
9.00 – 10.00	Breakfast got dressed **8**	Breakfast got dressed **6**
10.00 – 11.00	Read paper, phoned friend **7**	Took dog in garden **6**

Times	Monday	Tuesday	Wednesday	Thursday	Friday	Saturday	Sunday
7.00 – 8.00							
8.00 – 9.00							
9.00 – 10.00							
10.00 – 11.00							
11.00 – 12.00							
12.00 – 1.00							
1.00 – 2.00							
2.00 – 3.00							
3.00 – 4.00							
4.00 – 5.00							
5.00 – 6.00							
6.00 – 7.00							
7.00 – 8.00							
8.00 – 9.00							
Late evening and over night							

Note: Fatigue levels: 10 (highest fatigue) to 1 (lowest fatigue)

Reviewing your activity diaries

The most important aspect of an activity diary is learning from it. You may have already used diaries and not found them useful. They are only helpful if they enable you to understand more about how you are using your energy. Typically, there are two very different fatigue patterns in CFS/ME.

Pattern 1: Boom and bust (fluctuating levels of fatigue)

'Boom and bust' is the most common pattern where fatigue levels are fluctuating and we have already looked at this (see diagram on page 17). You may already be able to see the variation in your energy levels when you look at your diaries. Here are some different options for using your diaries when you have fluctuating levels of fatigue.

If you want to start to understand any patterns to your fatigue levels you can use colour coding. For example, marking all fatigue levels above 7 in blue and all fatigue levels below 5 in yellow, will illustrate more dramatically any patterns of boom and bust.

Another system you may find helpful is to mark all high energy activities in red, the medium energy activities in orange and the low energy activities in green, like traffic lights, to see if all your energy is going on just a few high energy activities. Also, marking all pleasurable activities in pink can show up if you are doing only activities that you feel you should do and leaving out activities that you enjoy.

Another good starting point is to ask yourself what struck you when filling in the diary. The main problems may be obvious – for example, large time periods spent on one activity. Managing activity is often about 'common sense solutions'. You may already be aware of what is not working but are stuck as to how to change this. People are often able to identify where they have pushed past their energy limits but find it difficult to stop doing this.

See if there are any patterns in each day – for example, all activity is in the morning and you are resting all afternoon. To reduce the boom and bust cycle you will need to focus on levelling out your activity throughout the day.

Remember one of the commonest problems in CFS/ME is the fact that when energy levels rise, people tend to increase their levels of activity by too much. This leads to increases in 'rebound fatigue'. Rebound fatigue is when you experience delayed fatigue as a direct result of doing an activity. Sometimes people know they are doing too much on their 'good days', but don't want to 'give in to' the condition, or they find it hard to change how they have always been. To get a baseline you are first looking to reduce the fluctuations in your fatigue to a more stable pattern, and then gradually to build up your levels of activity.

> **Useful questions to ask yourself:**
> • What have you found to be most difficult this week?
> • What do you feel may have triggered the worsening in your fatigue?
> • How could you have done things differently?

Pattern 2: Stuck in the mud (stable levels of fatigue)

Some people find that their fatigue levels are not changing. This may be because they have already limited their activity to avoid higher levels of fatigue, or sometimes the pattern has changed from previously fluctuating to now remaining around the same level.

If your fatigue levels have improved overall and now you seem stuck at around the same level all the time – for example, always scoring 6-7 out of 10 – then this may indicate that you have found your baseline. Now you need to start applying the grading strategies in the next section. Equally, you may have had some improvement before through grading and have now 'plateaued'. There is more information on dealing with plateaus in Chapter 10 on Relapses and Setbacks.

However, if you find your fatigue levels are so high – for example, always around 8-9 out of 10, even though you have restricted yourself to very low levels of activity – this can sometimes need a different approach. This is because you have not got any periods of relative 'over activity' to reduce – so where do you start?

With this pattern it is important to remember that the human body needs activity in order to produce energy. Limiting your activity can make you feel exhausted, lethargic and increase pain when you do move. Also, activity is needed to improve your mental skills, such as memory and concentration, and to maintain your confidence. Take the example of people who have been forced to be more inactive, such as in some reality TV shows. Over time their sleep cycle is disturbed and they have increased fatigue, lethargy, and sleep during the day.

As you grow up you may have been taught that when you are ill you need to rest. This is very important for helping the body to focus its energy on tackling acute health problems. However, having CFS/ME is not an acute health problem. You are probably reading this book because you expected the fatigue and other symptoms to resolve a long time ago. The problem with *only* resting over a longer period is that this starts to create problems in itself. Your body is designed to be *doing*, so if there is nothing to do, your body will not produce increased energy. So your fatigue and pain levels will increase as you are less mobile. Therefore this becomes a vicious circle, as illustrated in the next diagram.

This is a situation where you are fatigued if you do things and you are equally fatigued if you do not. Also, the less you do the more fed up and frustrated you feel, so your risk of becoming depressed will increase.

It is very difficult when you are stuck between the 'frying pan and the fire' and your fatigue is not reducing on its own. So you may have to work through the high levels of fatigue very gently, making tiny steps forward, very slowly increasing your levels of activity, despite your fatigue. In this case, you are aiming to

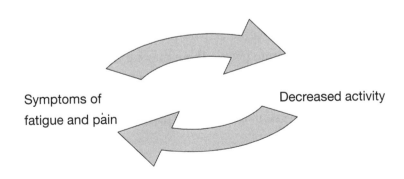

Symptoms of
fatigue and pain

Decreased activity

remain around the same level of fatigue and avoid making too big a step, which increases your fatigue further. This is very difficult to do and can feel like walking along the edge of a cliff, but if nothing else is helping it is sometimes the only way to get to the other side.

> **Useful questions to ask yourself:**
> - Has doing nothing or very little improved your fatigue?
> - What is likely to happen to your general health and your body if you stay inactive?
> - Obviously, if you do too much activity this can make the fatigue worse, but will doing a very small amount of activity make any difference?
> - What are the benefits of doing a little bit more, physically and psychologically?
> - If you are doing very little anyway, does it matter if you have to rest more so that you can do something you enjoy?

The helicopter view – seeing the bigger picture

Earlier we looked at how activity is complicated and how many different things can influence the way in which you live your life. Therefore, fatigue can be affected by a broad range of factors, not just how much energy you spend on each individual task. For many people focusing in detail on how they are using their energy, through using the activity recording method, helps them find somewhere to start. For some people there may be other key factors impacting on their fatigue, or this approach of analysing activity may not suit them. Therefore, in the next section we will look at another model for understanding energy before we look at how to change your daily life.

Supply and demand

Another way to understand the importance of grading and balancing activities is the concept of balancing scales. On one side of the scales is your energy supply, which is now much smaller than it was in the past. On the other side are all the demands on that energy.

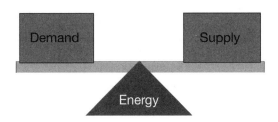

Improving supply

There may be things that you can do to help improve your supply of energy. For example, you may have looked at improving your diet or sleep, aspects of which are included in later chapters.

A helpful way to think about your energy supply is to think about an energy 'bank'. Inside your bank is your energy, which due to CFS/ME is now at a much lower level than before. Every day you give different amounts of your energy to all the things that your body and mind have to do. Some things will take more of your energy supply than others, for example fighting an infection or dealing with stress. There are other things in life that give you energy. The first things you might think of are food and sleep, but many other things can also do this. If you find something enjoyable or fun this can give you energy. If you feel you have achieved something or feel proud about something this can energise you. So, there are some activities that take energy to do, but you can also get some energy back from them.

When people get CFS/ME they often focus on the things they feel they *have* to do, like housework or sorting the bills. These are the activities from which you probably do not get any enjoyment or satisfaction, so put nothing back into the 'bank'. Whereas, activities that are seen as taking up energy, such as interests or time with friends, are the first to be sacrificed. Even though these activities maybe the things that help to top up your energy supply.

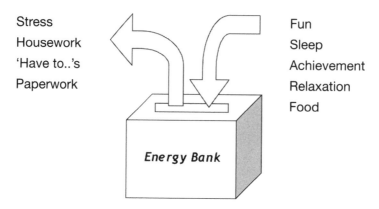

Stress	Fun
Housework	Sleep
'Have to..'s	Achievement
Paperwork	Relaxation
	Food

Decreasing demand

The demands on your energy can be both positive and negative, and come from lots of different sources, such as family, work, running a house, etc. They can also come from the pressure of trying to meet your own expectations or standards. It can therefore be helpful to identify whether any of these things could be done differently, whether anyone could help with these demands, or whether they need to be done at all!

Sometimes you may have demands that you can do nothing to change. If they really cannot be managed differently and if you do not have enough energy to do them all, then you might decide that your fatigue is not going to change until something else in the balance changes, such as your financial situation or support from others. The next exercise will help you to look at areas of supply or demand that you could work on.

> ## Task
> Make a list of the key things that help with the supply of your energy and the main areas of demand on your energy.

Demands	Supply

Useful questions to ask yourself:
- Look at the list of demands. Ask yourself if each one is absolutely necessary. What would happen if you did not do it?
- If you have to do them, can you prioritise them into an order so you can focus on one task at a time?
- Could anyone else help you with any of this – for example, getting financial advice or contacting a local support group?

Making changes - the principles of how to grade your activity

Once you have a more in-depth understanding of your current fatigue levels the next stage is to look at how you can influence these, through changing your daily patterns of activity. We previously explored how all activities are made up of component parts and each of those components requires energy. Therefore, some activities can be made easier by simply reducing the number of component parts involved. For example, if you do the ironing sitting down, you are not using the additional energy required to stand up. Activities can be made easier or harder depending on how you do them.

By understanding the different methods by which activity can be broken down, you can begin to understand the process of *grading*. The next section will describe the different ways in which activity can be broken into smaller parts, so that you can begin to grade what you are doing.

Breaking down activity - ways to grade

1. Time
The longer the period of time spent on an activity the more energy it will require. Time is the easiest way to measure what you are doing, and therefore

is the one used most often. You can set a baseline time limit for each activity – for example, reading for 10 minutes. Gradually increase the time periods allocated to each task, so the next step might be 11 minutes. The initial time period should be based on how long you can tolerate the activity for on a consistent basis without experiencing increased fatigue afterwards. (In the next section we will look more at when to stop.) Once this can be maintained the time period can be gradually increased for one activity at a time.

2. Distance

Distance is a more useful measure for any activity that involves motion, such as walking, swimming, driving etc. People can often be focused on reaching the destination, such as getting to the local shop, and find it difficult to stop before this point. It may be hard to see the purpose in walking only part of the way along the street, resting and returning. However, by doing this slowly and consistently you can build up the amount that you can walk. The aim is that you can get to the shop once you have built up to that distance. The most important thing is to identify markers for each distance so that you know how far you have gone and can measure improvement. For example, you can use lamp posts on a street or benches on a walk in the park.

3. Speed

Speed is the combination of time and distance, the ability to perform the task faster. It is often the case with fatigue that 'more haste makes less speed'. When people hurry an activity they will make a higher number of mistakes and often experience increased fatigue following the activity. Some people with CFS/ME would have done activities at a fast pace in the past, so they would think fast, walk fast and talk fast. Even though you have fatigue, when you have the energy to do any mental or physical activity you may still do it at a fast pace. Therefore, the first step is to *reduce* the speed at which you do things. Increasing speed is not a useful focus for grading until the final stage of your recovery.

4. Strength

This relates to muscle power and stamina. Muscle bulk decreases through in-activity. People who have previously maintained high levels of physical activity may be frustrated by the effects of muscles becoming de-conditioned. Strength can be regained in response to the demands of an activity only through gradu-ally increasing the muscle power needed for the task. To grade any activity requiring strength, make the load involved as light as possible to start with and then gradually increase it. Some examples might be: for arms, gradually increas-ing the amount of weight carried in shopping bags; for legs, this might involve slowly increasing the number of stairs you are climbing.

5. Resistance

Resistance is related to strength. The more resistance encountered the more strength is required to complete the activity. It is important when you are trying to make tasks easier that resistance is reduced wherever possible. An example is walking along level ground to start with, rather than up a hill.

6. Rest

People often use the word 'rest' to refer to when they are sitting or lying down. However, you can still be using mental or physical energy in these positions – for example, watching TV. This is therefore not 'rest'. It is important to think about 'quality' rest, when you really relax and let your battery recharge. **How you rest is as important as the activity you do** Prolonged periods of rest increase your physical de-conditioning.

As the joints become stiff and the muscles weaken, it requires a greater amount of energy to start activity again. Therefore, it is important to use rest as a pause within activity for the body to relax, but to try to avoid long periods of inactivity. If you currently choose to complete an activity all in one go before your 'energy runs out', you may find that by switching between short periods of activity and rest you can increase the total amount of activity you can complete.

7. Complexity

Complexity is an issue most associated with mental tasks. The more processes that are required to complete the task, the more energy it will need. People who are fatigued can lose the ability to concentrate on different activities at the same time - for example, talking on the telephone and remembering a message. Therefore, to make tasks easier they need to be simplified. So it helps if you can **focus on one task at a time** and reduce all distractions, such as background noise.

The dangers of the 'starter-finisher'

Some people have always lived by the rule that when they start a job they have to keep going until it's finished. They find it very difficult to stop an activity in progress. This works well when your energy is there so you can get to the finish. However, for people with CFS/ME often the energy has run out part way through and they find they are pushing their bodies to try to get to the end, like driving the car on the empty fuel light. This then reinforces the 'boom and bust' pattern. Often this also results in people not starting any activities they want to do because they know they will not be able to finish them.

There is another way, which follows the story of the tortoise and the hare. Instead of racing to get to the end of the task and having to rest, like the hare, you can take the tortoise approach of taking small slow steps. It might be slower, which is frustrating, but by a steady approach you can get to the end of the job.

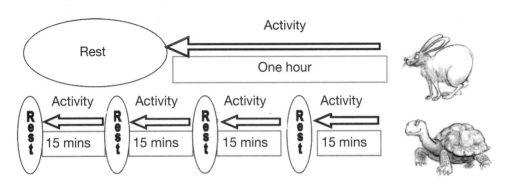

Take the example of an hour of housework. If you do this now with CFS/ME you might have to stop and give up after 30 minutes, or keep putting it off until you have a 'good' day and can face doing it. If you did 15 minutes at four times spread through the day then you might manage it.

Setting your stopping point

One problem you may have is knowing when to stop an activity. Often people with CFS/ME do not stop until they are beginning to experience significant increases in their symptoms. If you rely on our body to tell you when to stop you will already have done too much.

A helpful way to understand this is to think about the braking distance for cars. In this situation, if the car needs to stop to prevent it hitting a wall, then the brakes need to be applied with enough time for the car to slow down. This avoids damage being done to the car. In the same way, the body needs to stop before you hit the wall, not after you have started to feel the effects.

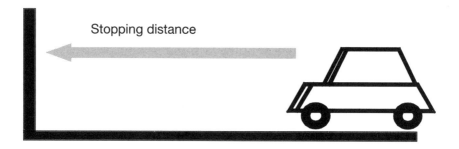

Stopping distance

Unfortunately the body has no indicators for when to stop and so the braking distance for each person can be found only through trial and success. You can experiment with your stopping distance only if you are measuring what you are doing in the first place. Then you know when you might hit the wall and, from that, set a time or distance, etc, to stop before you do this. You will then have to test this out a few times to check if this is the right point for you to manage consistently. This is because you may have been having a good day or there may be a longer delay in your fatigue than you thought.

The next task will focus you on how to start breaking down an activity and finding the point at which you should stop. If you can get this right with one activity you can then apply the same method to the other things that you do.

Task

Select one activity that you would like to be able to undertake on a regular basis.

- How could you break this down into manageable steps using one or more of the approaches that have been described?
- How are you going to measure each step?
- Write a plan for this week that includes the first step for your activity. Think about whether this needs to be done every day or at intervals through the week. Is there a best time of the day to do it? Are you going to need any help?
- Do your first step and record what happens. It may help to write down your fatigue level, using the scale of 0–10 again, before, during and after the activity to know more about its impact. If there is a significant increase in your fatigue, reduce your planned stopping point for the next time you repeat it.

Keep repeating the process each time you do the activity until you find a level that does not significantly increase your fatigue afterwards.

For example:

Date	Activity/ Task	Stopping point (time/distance/etc)	Result
Wed 4/3	Reading the paper	10 mins	Before 5, During 5, After 6. Try 8 mins
Fri 6/3	Reading the paper	8 mins	Before 6, During 6, After 6. Repeat 8 mins next time

Date	Activity/ Task	Stopping point (time/distance/etc)	Result

Combining activities

We do not undertake activities in isolation. Our day contains a varied combination of tasks, each with its own physical, mental and social demands. Therefore, how each activity interacts with the others within our day is vitally important. It is crucial to maintain a balance across the activities in your day so that activities with a high level of similar demand are not grouped together, increasing fatigue.

Mix and match

Mixing and matching different types of activities within your day can help to maintain energy levels, as some parts of your body can relax whilst others are working. A general rule is to set up a routine for yourself that involves short periods of different types of activity. For example, changing between physical, mental and social activities and rest periods can be used to maximise the energy that you have or to prevent increasing fatigue levels.

The idea is not to do two things in a row that are similar. An example would be reading and then filling in a form, which are both mental activities. Remember you may have different tolerances for different activities, such as for mental or physical tasks, so think about the stopping point for each one separately, based on what suits you.

For example:

Time	Activity	Type of activity
10.00	Washing up (10 mins)	Physical
10.10	Rest / relaxation (20 mins)	Rest
10.30	Read paper (15 mins)	Mental

10.45	Phone a friend (15 mins)	Social
11.00	Rest / relaxation (20 mins)	Rest
11.20	Watched TV (30 mins)	Mental

Incorporating pleasure

People who have CFS/ME often feel guilty about not doing the jobs that they think they should do, or are expected to do. So when they have any energy they push themselves to do activities that they feel they 'have to do' and sacrifice pleasurable and fun activities. But things that you enjoy or give you a sense of achievement can give you energy, and therefore are another source of supply for your energy bank.

To help to understand this, think of the story of two men who run a race and they both finish the race in two hours, using up around the same amount of energy. For the first man, this is the worst time he has ever run and he feels exhausted and frustrated at his performance. It might take him some time to recover from the effort of the race. For the second man, this is the best time he has ever done. Although he feels fatigued he also feels elated and energised by his performance, and is likely to recover more quickly.

For this reason, sometimes even though you may feel fatigued by an activity it may also give you satisfaction, enjoyment and help you feel more positive. This can help to sustain you, which means that sometimes you might exceed your energy limits to do something you enjoy. Remember you will need to adjust your programme to allow for some additional rest, before and after a pleasurable activity. You may also need to reduce other activities to compensate for this.

Useful questions to ask yourself:
- What do I really enjoy or look forward to each week?
- Are there things I used to do but no longer do, because I would feel guilty about wasting energy on these?
- How did my fatigue feel the last time I did something I enjoyed?

Task

Make a list of things that you are currently able to do that you enjoy or help you to feel relaxed. Add any activities that you think you could manage but have not been doing for other reasons.

Think about how you could incorporate these within your routine.

Making the grade

We have discussed before the importance of being able both to pace and to grade your activity. The word 'grading' means to arrange in degrees and to reduce to easy gradients (*Oxford English Dictionary*, 1998). This is different to 'pacing', which means to set the pace or measure for a distance. The difference between pacing and grading is that setting a pace or speed for activities is an important part of setting a baseline for fatigue, and grading implies movement or progression through levels of activity. Therefore, finding your starting point and stabilising your fatigue levels is only the first step in managing fatigue. This can take a long time, but once you have achieved this you can start to focus on building up what you can do. There is no set formula for each increase, in the same way as the starting point is different for everyone. We cannot just say, for example, increase each activity by five minutes each week, as this does not take account of how you respond to each increase and whether this is too big a step for you.

It is important to understand that the pattern of grading activity is like a staircase, not a slope. Whenever an increase in activity is made, this level needs to be maintained before another increase is added. This is important as the condition often has a fluctuating pattern. If you make increases during periods of improved energy, then you cannot keep this going when your energy levels reduce. This can increase the 'boom and bust' effect.

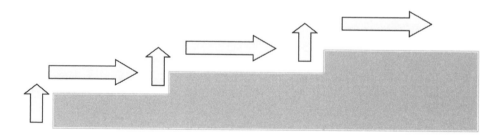

Make each increase small enough so that it is not so different to your current level that your body then reacts – for example, only increasing by around 10 per cent of what you currently can manage. Better to make more small steps initially, than one big one, crash and give up. As you improve, your steps are likely to become bigger, but it is important to be realistic at the beginning.

Remember, if you are physically doing slightly more you may get some reaction initially. This will also occur when someone who is well starts to exercise for the first time or increase their activity levels. They may feel great immediately afterwards, but may not be able to walk the next day! You will need to work out the difference between the signs that you have done more than normal and an increase in your fatigue symptoms, which is not easy to do. You need to understand and work together with your body.

What if it goes wrong?

A graded approach is about taking a slow and steady approach to improvement in your symptoms. However, as CFS/ME has a fluctuating pattern it can still feel like a rollercoaster at times. Through using this method you may find that when you have a relapse you may initially go back a few steps, but usually you do not tumble down to the bottom. Chapter 10 is designed to help you to deal with 'Relapse and Setbacks'.

If someone has a significant relapse, such as having a bad virus, bereavement or additional stress, they often report that the symptoms improve again quicker than they did before if they have been following a more consistent approach. You may have to start at a lower activity level again but you can work back to where you were.

If you are struggling with grading or find you have got stuck on one level, which can often be described as 'plateauing', think about other things stopping you from making progress. Information on dealing with some of the typical things that can also affect symptoms is talked about in other chapters. Remember, there are also health professionals who can help you with this approach and you can discuss how to get more help with your general practitioner (GP).

Useful resources

- Cox DL (2000) *Occupational Therapy and Chronic Fatigue Syndrome.* London: Whurr
- Thew M, Pemberton S (2008) Energy for Life. In: Thew M, McKenna J (Eds) *Lifestyle Management in Health and Social Care.* Chichester: Blackwell Publishing

Catherine's story

I started experiencing the symptoms of CFS/ME in June 1998. By 2006, I was stuck in a cycle of being active in the mornings, then going to bed exhausted and sleeping for between two and three hours every afternoon. I would get up again in the late afternoon and manage some further light activity in the evenings, before going to bed again. My sleep was often disturbed and I would wake several times a night. My main symptoms were fatigue, muscle pain, especially in my thighs, migraine, blurred vision and digestive problems. I was aware that I often tried to take on too many things and even tried to ignore my illness. I continued to push myself every day. I would make unrealistic lists of the tasks I wanted to complete and I would overstretch myself. Then, often I would end up feeling that I had not achieved anything and that I never did very much. I felt that my life was restricted by the illness.

I had not been able to increase my energy levels by myself. I had been unable to break my routine of cramming all my activity into the mornings and then collapsing into bed with exhaustion after lunch. I identified with the boom and bust method of coping. I realised that managing my activities every day would increase my activity levels over a period of time, which was exactly what I was struggling with.

When I began incorporating these management strategies into my life, I did not know how much activity I could manage before it caused my fatigue levels to increase. Every day I would stop only when I could not continue any longer. Then my physical or mental fatigue was so severe, that I was forced to go to bed and sleep. My first task was, therefore, to work out how much I could manage to do before it increased my symptoms.

I accepted that I needed to spread my limited energy over the whole day: do less than I was doing in the mornings, so that I still had some energy left in the afternoons and evenings. I found that by completing activity diaries everyday for several weeks I began to see which activities caused my fatigue levels to rise. It also made me think about how I was spending my time: how much time I was spending doing chores and jobs which I felt needed doing, and how much time I was spending doing things that gave me pleasure and which I enjoyed. At the start I felt that completing activity diaries was tedious, boring and even a waste of time! However, I realised that if I wrote down every hour how I had spent my time and what my fatigue level was on a scale of 1 to 10 during that hour, they could be a useful tool. I saw that time spent resting and relaxing was just as important as time spent 'doing'. By taking regular shorter rests throughout the day I could make my energy last for longer. I accepted that because I was sleeping for a fairly long period every day I should start by first cutting down the amount of sleep I was having in the afternoons. I did not cut it out completely to begin with because I felt that it would be too big a step to take all at once.

I learned about the concept of the human battery: how by always keeping going until my battery was completely empty of energy before I stopped, I was never leaving any energy spare for recovery and healing. I could see that the way that I had been managing my symptoms was not leaving any energy available for rest and recovery. Initially, I felt that the effort and thought that were involved in following the advice seemed hard work. It also actually put more restrictions on my life, because it stopped me from doing just what I wanted to do, when I wanted to do it. However, I soon realised that by being disciplined and following the advice, I could begin to see some positive results. This made me feel more in control of my illness. My improvement was slow and I needed to commit to the approach and stick at it over a period of time.

There is no quick fix to the problem of CFS/ME. However, I was motivated to keep going, even though I did not always get it right, because I realised that I could actually have some control over how I felt.

One approach that I found useful was switching between different types of activities frequently. I would previously have started a task, such as doing paperwork, and continued with it until it was finished or until fatigue prevented me from continuing. Then I would be forced to go to bed to sleep. I had no idea that if I spent half an hour doing paperwork, then stopped and lay down on the sofa, practised relaxation techniques for 15 minutes, spent half an hour ironing, then made a drink and sat down for 10 minutes - that I could then spend another half an hour doing paperwork and still feel reasonably ok. Previously I would have spent an hour doing paperwork, with little or no break, and then have felt absolutely exhausted at the end of it. I have found that taking mini breaks and switching between different activities does work.

By following the advice I have come to realise that some activities actually give me energy. If I am doing something which I really enjoy I automatically feel better. This may seem surprisingly simply and obvious. Until it was actually pointed out to me, I did not fully understand that I could improve my energy levels just by looking forward to something and enjoying an activity. I also had not realised that even in healthy people energy levels fluctuate throughout the day. Often people will 'switch off' and relax without really thinking about it but I was someone who had previously ignored these natural slumps. I had kept pushing myself even when I did not feel up to it.

I also realised that simple, and again not obvious, things could make the task easier and use less energy. For example, sitting at the kitchen table to prepare vegetables for dinner rather than standing at the worktop. I started doing things more slowly than I had previously. I made conscious decisions to walk more slowly, even to think more slowly. Although tasks took longer, I did not collapse with exhaustion at the end of them as I once had and I still had some energy left.

I learned not to use that remaining energy to accomplish another task and to stop and rest before my body forced me to stop.

Also, I realised that I had to work at not pushing myself too hard and feeling disappointed when I failed to complete what I had started. I learned to be more honest with myself about what I could do and to plan realistic amounts of activities. If I finished a task quicker than I had expected to, I would use the rest of the time I had allocated to that task to rest and relax.

Gradually I understood that what I had been doing before was not working for me and that I had been stuck in a cycle of boom and bust. I began to understand that I could move forward and that what I was learning could bring improvement to my health. The tasks that I completed helped me by making me really think about what I had been doing. How everything, even the things that I had considered to be automatic, such as getting out of bed in the morning or making a cup of tea, use energy and therefore affect fatigue. The level of detail and analysis that I felt I had to go into did initially feel laborious and even a little unnecessary for me, as I was used just to getting on with things. However, I eventually realised that many different factors can have a significant impact on my energy levels. Even the seemingly simplest of tasks are often very complicated and when my body was not functioning as it used to, even those simple tasks were difficult to carry out.

I began to feel more in control of how I was feeling and know that if I followed the advice, I could improve my energy levels and symptoms.

Chapter Two

Rest

Sue Pemberton

Introduction

People often talk about using rest when referring to problems with fatigue, but what do we mean by rest? Is resting a good or bad approach to managing your symptoms? This chapter will explore the value of quality rest and the common problems that people can experience with rest. Please complete the sheet below to help you as you read through the chapter.

Summary sheet

Topic	Read	Comments
Self-assessment		
What is rest?		
Stopping what you are doing		
Allowing yourself to rest		

Staying in one position		
Achieving quality rest – test yourself		

Self-assessment

Everyone thinks about and experiences 'rest' in different ways, so it is important to start by reflecting on your own views of rest. Think about your answers to the following questions and then you will be able to reflect on these when we get to the end of the chapter.

Task

- In what ways do you rest now?

- What did you think about the idea of resting before you became ill?

- How do you feel about yourself and your life while you are resting?

What is rest?

The *Concise Oxford English Dictionary* (2006) defines 'to rest' as:

- cease work or movement in order to relax or recover strength
- allow to be inactive in order to regain or save strength or energy
- place or be placed so as to stay in a specified position: *his feet rested on the table.*

We are going to look at all of these aspects of rest in relation to your CFS/ME.

Stopping what you are doing

The first definition of rest describes ceasing or stopping activity. Most people will say that they *have* to rest because they come to the point where they just can't continue with activity. This can result in them having to rest for long periods of time. However, the definition goes on to say 'in order to relax or recover strength'. Therefore, relaxation and recovery are the purpose of resting. However, *stopping* physical activity and *relaxing* are not necessarily the same thing. For example, if you have stopped physically moving but are lying there thinking about the things that you should be doing, or feeling irritated that you have had to stop, you will not feel relaxed. So for many people, the quality of their rest is very poor as they may spend many hours inactive but, without knowing it, are inhibiting the body's ability to use rest to recover energy.

Also, people who develop CFS/ME tend to have been very active before they were ill. They are not used to stopping activity and therefore they are more likely to find rest frustrating and 'a waste of time'. This means there is a high chance that resting is not going to be a relaxing experience. To many people in western cultures a lack of overt activity can be seen as 'nothing is happening'. However, in other cultures around the world the periods between activities are seen as equally valuable as the activity itself. In China, for example, waiting or 'non activity' is viewed as an important step before activity to help it to be meaningful.

Some people may feel uncomfortable stopping activity altogether. As the purpose of rest is to relax, some people may actually get more benefit from doing a gentle activity that they find relaxing, rather than stopping activity completely. You may be someone who finds reading a book, talking to friends or watching a film relaxing and that these help increase your energy. Or you may be someone for whom these activities are draining. So it is important to change your thinking about rest from 'stopping activity altogether' to focusing on the best ways for you to relax.

Useful questions to ask yourself:
- In what ways do I relax now?
- How can I improve the quality of my rest so that I find it more relaxing?

Allowing yourself to rest

A big problem for many people with CFS/ME is that they know they should rest/relax more, but they do not actually do this in their daily life. There can be lots of thoughts that stop you from allowing yourself to relax. Common thoughts can include:

- 'Resting is a waste of time.'
- 'Because I am not able to do all the things I should do each day, I have to keep going while I can.'
- 'If I rest it is giving into to the condition.'
- 'If I rest it is hard for me to get going again afterwards.'
- 'I only rest when I have to.'
- 'I never used to have to rest, so I don't see why I should now.'

- 'Too many people depend on me.'
- 'Other people can't see that I am ill and so will think poorly of me if I have to rest.'
- 'My doctor told me to rest all the time but that just makes me feel worse.'

These thoughts can be very powerful as they can stop you from doing something that you know could help your health. Many people with CFS/ME report that they carried on doing a task even though they knew that they should stop and rest. If you don't tackle these beliefs, nothing will change - regardless of how many pages we write about the benefits of rest!

Here are some ideas for challenging these beliefs, but you may be able to come up with other alternatives that you can relate to.

- **Resting is a waste of time** – so you believe either that your recovery isn't important or that rest doesn't have any benefits? If the doctor told you to take a tablet every four hours that would help you and you have to rest for 30 minutes after taking it, you would probably do this. So if the doctor prescribes short periods of rest without the tablet, would you do it? Relaxing changes the physiological responses in our bodies. It activates the parasympathetic nervous system, which enables us to digest food, supports our immune system and generates energy supplies. All of the processes it carries out are necessary for your body to function. Does maintaining your body's systems and producing energy supplies sound like 'a waste of time'?

- **Because I am not able to do all the things I should do each day, I have to keep going while I can** - Pushing yourself to be as active as you can be (when the energy is there) will keep re-enforcing the 'boom-bust' pattern of your CFS/ME. This may give you short term reward rather than long term gain. So you might get more things done on one day, but it will not help you improve your overall fatigue levels or promote recovery. You can still achieve as much in total by pacing out your activity (with rest in-between) as you can doing it all in one go - sometimes you may even achieve more. Think about the example from Chapter 1 that doing an hour's work followed by an hour's rest is the same as doing 4 x 15 minutes of work, with 15 minutes' rest after each one. Think about how you would feel after doing an hour of an activity compared with just doing 15 minutes of it. It is much more likely that you would be able to keep going for longer taking small regular rests than using the 'all at once' approach.

- **If I rest it is giving in to the condition** - People often fear that if they stop pushing themselves, then they will be letting the condition take over. 'Giving in to the condition' is a state of mind, rest is a physiological process - the two do not necessarily have any connection. For example, an athlete may use rest/relaxation as a positive part of her preparations for a race. This does not mean she does not want to win the race; it means she wants her muscles to be in the best possible condition for when they are needed. It is important to separate out the idea of rest from any concerns you have about giving up on life. Any worries about the illness need to be addressed separately. Remember, if you have always been a fighter in life it is unlikely that taking some rest is going to change that.

- **If I rest it is hard for me to get going again afterwards** - Initiating movement and activity after long periods of rest or sleep can be very difficult. When the body is still for a period of time the muscles and joints may tighten. This may cause more pain or stiffness when you start trying to move again. If you have been dozing or sleeping during a rest period it may take time to feel mentally alert again. If this is a real problem for you it may help to change *how* you are resting. The longer the rest, the more difficult it is likely to be to get moving again. Think about having much shorter rest periods, but more frequently. Even taking a minute out to slow your breathing and relax your body can have benefits. Also, think about the position in which you rest; if you are likely to fall asleep resting on the bed, relax in a chair. Higher chairs are easier to get up from afterwards, so this may help if you get pain or stiffness.

- **I only rest when I have to** - When you get to the point that your only option is to rest, you have gone too far. It is important to use rest to help prevent the increase in symptoms, not just to recover from them. What if you only ate when you were really starving? That would not be the healthiest approach for your body. In the same way, only resting when you absolutely have to is not helping your body to function at its best. The saying goes 'work, rest and play' for a reason. Rest is an important part of your body's system for maintaining health. Many people with CFS/ME eat a healthy diet, not because they believe it will cure their fatigue, but because they know it will help their body to function most effectively. Taking *'healthy rest'* as a positive strategy is just as important.

- **I never used to have to rest, so I don't see why I should now** - You did not have CFS/ME before! The way you did things before you became ill may not help you now. Doing things differently now and using rest between activities may help you to recover.

- **Too many people depend on me** - You cannot help others in the way you would like to if you are feeling so ill. The best way to help them is to improve your health. Also, many people do not learn to do things for themselves if they have someone else to do it for them. This might be an opportunity for them to start taking responsibility for themselves. If you were not around what would they do?

- **Other people can't see that I am ill and so will think poorly of me if I have to rest** - How are they going to understand that you are unwell if they never see the consequences of this, such as your taking more rest?

Which is more important - their opinion of you or doing what you need to do to get better? Sometimes they might be glad that you have suggested taking a rest because they wanted to, but did not want to admit this to you!

- **My doctor told me to rest all the time but that just makes me feel worse** - Rest and relaxation are important when the body needs to deal with an acute health problem, such as an infection or injury. This is because relaxation helps to trigger the right nervous system response to enable your immune system to function, supports growth and regeneration in the body, and conserves energy. So, often a health professional may advise rest in the early stages of the condition or in response to a relapse. However, resting for a prolonged period of time can have negative effects on the body as human beings are designed to be active. The next section will look at the problems of resting too much.

Useful questions to ask yourself:
- What stops me from taking more regular rest?
- How am I going to change this so that I use 'healthy rest' as part of my recovery?

Staying in one position

Many people think that resting is keeping physically still, so that sitting or lying in one position is an important part of rest. As we have already observed, it is whether we are relaxed that is the important part of rest, which may involve staying physically still or it may not. However, staying inactive for long periods does start to have effects on the body and it is important to be aware of this.

In just the same way that overdoing activity can increase your symptoms of CFS/ME, so can continuing levels of 'under activity', where we are doing only minimal levels of movement. Chapter 9 on 'Physical Activity and Exercise' describes what can happen to the body with prolonged under activity, including: decreased muscle efficiency and increased muscle contraction; changes in blood pressure and the deconditioning of blood vessels; decreased bone calcium; impairment of nerve function; disruption of regulatory functions (such as sleep hormones, or temperature control); and lower cortisol levels.

Our bodies are designed to move, so it is important to keep making small amounts of movement, to maintain the ability to function. Therefore, having smaller amounts of rest between periods of activity is physiologically better than taking long periods. Even if you are confined to bed, it is important to change your position of rest regularly. For example, changing between lying down and sitting up supported by pillows can help to maintain blood pressure, and joint flexibility.

Your body also does not think it needs to generate energy if there is no demand. Remember, bears hibernate in the winter because there is nothing to do, as there is little food to hunt and they need to conserve energy. Often when people are made to do very little or are kept in confined places, they will start to feel increased levels of fatigue and may start to sleep more.

Posture during rest is also important. When you are resting try to avoid sitting or lying in positions where one muscle group is held tight, such as lying curled up in a ball or sitting hunched up. You want to allow all of the muscles in your body the chance to relax.

Achieving quality rest – test yourself

- Rest is not just the 'absence of doing'. To achieve quality rest you need to see it as a positive strategy that helps your body to access its natural systems for regeneration and recovery.

When you answered the questions at the beginning of this chapter, what did you believe about the importance of rest?
Mark yourself on this scale:
Waste of time--------------------------------Highly important

How would you rate this now?
Waste of time--------------------------------Highly important

- Give yourself a 'prescription' for rest. Decide how often and in what way you can rest within your daily life. Remember, just as with a healthy diet, the more frequently you stick to it the better the results.

How much rest do you feel you currently take, on a daily basis?

Too little ☐   Too much ☐   Just right ☐
How much total rest would you like to achieve each day? ☐

- Keep it balanced with activity. There may be times when you need to increase the amount of rest you take but keeping it balanced with periods of activity is important. Go for small and often if you can.

How are you going to improve the balance in your day between work, rest and play? I can improve my balance by…..

- The aim is to relax, so that involves your mind as well as your body.

I can make my rest more relaxing by….

Useful resources

- Chalder T (1995) *Coping with Chronic Fatigue Syndrome.* London: Sheldon Press
- Cox DL (2000) *Occupational Therapy and Chronic Fatigue Syndrome.* London: Whurr
- Chambers (2006) *Concise English Dictionary.* Edinburgh: Chambers Harrap Publishers
- Levine R (2006) *A Geography of Time – the temporal misadventures of a social psychologist.* Oxford: One World Publications

Mary's story

I became ill 10 years ago. For the first three months or so, I could not do much other than lie on the sofa. In time, I began to regain some energy, to the degree that now I am moderately affected by CFS/ME.

Before becoming ill I do not recall thinking much about rest, except in the context of my busy life, by looking for ways to make one day each week more restful than the other six. As I began facing up to having CFS/ME, I started learning about pacing and other management strategies. As part of pacing, I incorporated several rest periods into my daily routine.

Some years after the onset of my CFS/ME, I heard about some relaxation classes that had started up. I only made it to three out of the six classes but this was enough to transform the way I used my rest time.

I now believe that rest is one of the keys to my recovery from CFS/ME. I think my recovery could be further on if I were able to put into practice with more consistency the things I have learned about rest. When I was first ill, I viewed rest as a nuisance and a waste of time. I have gradually embraced it as a healing, enhancing and essential part of my life.

The key for me is to relax my muscles as much as possible, as well as my mind. There are relaxation techniques which help me to do that. I focus on my breathing and body and include visualisation and affirming self-talk.

Over the years I have been given various relaxation tapes and CDs and I have found some of them helpful. I learned abdominal breathing early in my illness and have built on that foundation. I benefited greatly from attending a relaxation group and the training it gave me.

I practise relaxation techniques daily, sometimes listening to a tape of these. As I do my relaxation, I often find that I need to keep bringing my thoughts back to the routine when I notice them wandering.

By learning and practising muscle relaxation, I have discovered tensions I was not aware of in my facial expression, limbs and back muscles, all of which I have learned consciously to let go. I now realise I can be lying still but not be relaxed. I also know it is possible to fall asleep with my muscles still tense, and wake up in pain.

I do a few gentle stretches before resting, to aid my muscles' relaxation. Taking appropriate levels of relaxing exercise during the day also helps my rest to be restful. For me, relaxing exercise means a few minutes stroll enjoying the fresh air, noticing my surroundings, swinging my arms, as opposed to a tense hurried walk of the same duration spent thinking about the other things I feel I ought to be doing.

My muscles instinctively tense up when I am cold. When I am cold I notice that I feel more ill and I benefit from being warm. I notice my symptoms of fatigue and muscle pain are less when I am warm and so I may use a hot water bottle during rests.

Anxiety increases my muscle tension and I find it difficult to relax my muscles when they are tense owing to the thoughts I am having. However, I am now sometimes able to shift a tension headache using self-talk and relaxation exercises and it is one step on the way to being in control of my symptoms.

Chapter Three

Sleep

Ian Portlock

Introduction

Difficulty with sleep is common for people with CFS/ME. Some people find they are sleeping too much, while others find they are not sleeping enough. If you experience problems with sleep there are several things you can do to help yourself.

There is no such thing as an ideal amount of sleep. For example, some people need 10 hours, while others need only five. An average night's sleep is around eight hours. When the amount of sleep someone is getting is causing an increase in fatigue that is when it becomes a problem.

When people first have CFS/ME they often over sleep. Suggestions as to what might be helpful if you are over sleeping are covered in the first part of this chapter. People who have had CFS/ME for a longer period of time often go from over sleeping to not being able to sleep enough, despite high fatigue levels. Suggestions that you might find helpful if you are not sleeping enough will be covered in the second part of the chapter.

This chapter provides a number of strategies for you to try, some of which you may find helpful, others you may not. Try these suggestions and remember that you can get further help with sleep problems from a health professional.

The summary sheet will help you to keep track of the sections of the chapter you have read and the sleep checklist at the end of the chapter will help you to record which strategies you found beneficial.

Summary sheet

Topic	Read	Comments
The sleep cycle		
Sleep diary		
Are you sleeping too much?		
Are you not sleeping enough?		
Adjusting your sleep pattern		
Summary		
Sleep checklist		

The sleep cycle

Most of the time we do not think about how we sleep; it is only when we start to have problems with our sleep that it begins to concern us. There are many common myths about sleep, such as: 'it is important to have eight hours every night'; 'broken sleep means poor quality sleep'; 'you should feel refreshed when you wake up because you have recharged your battery'; and 'if I could sleep better it would cure my fatigue'. However, understanding how sleep is structured, known as the 'architecture of sleep', can help to reduce some of the anxieties that may arise when we are not sleeping well.

The idea that you fall asleep, sleep solidly through the night and wake in the morning is misleading. Sleep is actually divided into five stages. These are Rapid Eye Movement (R.E.M.) sleep and stages 1, 2, 3, and 4. In R.E.M. sleep, the eyes move quickly behind the lids and it is the stage of sleep when dreaming occurs. As you sleep you descend through the stages, from R.E.M. to stage 4, which is the deepest form of sleep.

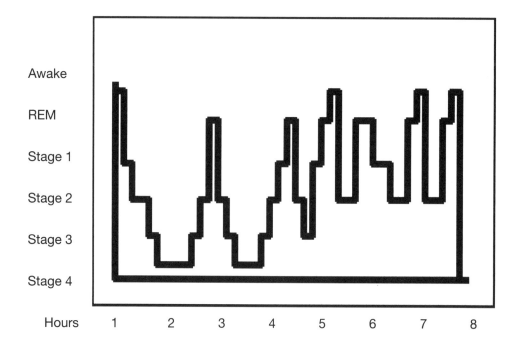

Throughout the night you move through the five stages of sleep a number of times. This pattern is called the 'sleep cycle'. One sleep cycle is roughly one and a half hours long. In the initial sleep cycle the majority of the time is spent in deep stage 4 sleep. In the successive sleep cycles that follow, an increasing amount of time is spent in R.E.M. and stage 2 sleep and a decreasing amount of time is spent in deep sleep.

The vast majority of deep sleep occurs within the first four hours. So in theory a healthy person who sleeps only four hours could get roughly the same amount of deep sleep as a person who sleeps for 12 hours a night. So when you have CFS/ME, it may be helpful to think about the sleep pattern you had before you were ill. You may have always been someone who needed more sleep or you may have functioned on less sleep. This may help when thinking about the sleep pattern you are aiming to achieve now.

Sleep diary

Why keep a sleep diary?

A sleep diary helps to evaluate your sleep problems. There are several reasons for doing this:

1. Keeping a sleep diary allows you to find out exactly what your current sleep pattern is, to help you to establish a baseline. For example, you may find you are getting more sleep than you thought.
2. The more you understand your sleep difficulties and your sleep patterns, the less anxious you will feel about them.
3. Keeping a diary will enable you to monitor your progress over time.

How to use the sleep diary

If you think it might be helpful, fill in the diary sheet provided in this chapter. Record your answers to the questions in the boxes provided. It is often best to answer the questions when you get up in the morning, before you forget and become occupied with the activities of the day.

Example of a completed sleep diary

Questions	Monday
Went to bed at	10.30 pm
Turned the light out at	11.15 pm
Fell asleep at	12.00 (approx)
Number of times sleep was interrupted	2
For how long	30 min and 20 min
Woke up at	8.00 am
Got up at	9.00 am
Fatigue level on waking	6
Overall sleep was	Restless/reasonable
Time spent 'catnapping' during day	10 min
Number of hours' sleep overall	7 hr 20 min

Task

Complete the sleep diary on the next page over the period of a week. Then review your answers to help you to know more about your current sleep pattern:
- How variable are the times that you are asleep?
- Is there anything that surprised you?
- What do you think are the main areas to address that might improve your sleep?

Are you sleeping too much?

When you have an acute illness, like an infection, your body may require more sleep to assist recovery. With CFS/ME, the fatigue and other symptoms are not improved by sleep so, although sleep may have been helpful at the beginning of your illness, it may not be making any difference now.

It is not unusual for people suffering from CFS/ME to report that they sleep for 12 or more hours, yet still feel fatigued and unrefreshed on waking. So with CFS/ME, on the odd occasion when you also have an acute illness or are sleep deprived, it is normal to 'catch up on sleep' by sleeping for longer than usual. However, some people with CFS/ME find that they regularly sleep much more than they did prior to the illness.

Often people think that if they are fatigued they need sleep, but the fatigue in CFS/ME is not improved by sleep. Therefore it is difficult for people to tell the difference between when they are tired due to lack of sleep and when they feel fatigued, which can be made worse by increased sleep.

The consequences of sleeping too much are:
- Increased need for more sleep.
- The body gets used to excessive sleep and late waking.
- Inability to concentrate properly.
- Loss of motivation and energy whilst awake.
- Reduced enjoyment and satisfaction with life.

Sleep diary

Week commencing:

Questions	Day 1	Day 2	Day 3	Day 4	Day 5	Day 6	Day 7
Went to bed at.....							
Turned light out at...							
Fell asleep at...							
Number of times sleep was interrupted...							
For how long.....							
Woke up at....							
Got up at.....							
Fatigue level on waking....							
Overall sleep was.....							
Time spent catnapping.....							
Number of hours sleep overall...							

What can you do practically about over sleeping?

First, complete the sleep diary to establish exactly how much sleep you are getting. If you are sleeping too much, look at *gradually* reducing your amount of sleep by getting up earlier. Aim to get up at the same time every morning and go to bed when you feel tired at night. When you have established a regular routine gradually reduce how long you are sleeping, for example by 15 minutes at a time. Establishing a routine will help you gain more control over your symptoms.

• Sleep routine
Everybody has a biological clock which regulates activity levels, temperature and sleep. The example of jet lag demonstrates how our body's rhythm can be out of synch with that of our environment. In CFS/ME some people will be sleeping in the day and be awake at night. Others will be 'cat napping' throughout the day.

• 'Catnapping'
It is advised that people with CFS/ME avoid 'cat napping' in the day if possible. 'Catnapping' can lead to people over sleeping or not being able to sleep at night. Also, many people feel groggy after sleeping and take a while to come round, often feeling worse than they did before they went to sleep. It is important in CFS/ME for people to balance the demands for energy that they are making on their body. This is difficult if your sleep routine is chaotic.

If you do not think you can manage to get through a whole day without sleeping, do not worry. Aim to regulate your sleep in the day to a particular time, e.g. 2 pm, and for a regular length, e.g. one hour. (An alarm clock may be needed to do this effectively.) Again, start with an amount of sleep that is similar to what your body is trying to take now. Once you have done this, reduce the amount of time you sleep during the day gradually over a few weeks, aiming eventually (if possible) to take all your sleep at night.

You may find it helpful, if you are used to 'catnapping', gradually to replace sleep during the day with quality rest. This allows you to help your body to recover when fatigued without disrupting your sleep pattern.

• Do not worry!
Initially the change to your sleeping pattern may make you feel worse and more fatigued. In the long term, you should feel more energised. Another benefit of reducing your sleep is that you will have more time available for the activities you choose to do.

> Quality not quantity also applies to sleep

If you do not manage to stop 'catnapping' or over sleeping completely, do not worry. Keep trying to regulate your sleep to the same time each day and reduce it as much as possible. Remember, altering your sleep pattern is important, but this is only one part of the management of CFS/ME.

Are you not sleeping enough?

Difficulty sleeping is common in CFS/ME. Do not panic if you are having trouble getting to sleep. One sleepless night has little effect on the body. Even if you have several bad nights, when you next fall asleep you will automatically catch up on deep sleep.

Here are some tips to help you manage lack of sleep:

• Wake up at a regular time
The time you wake up helps you to set your body clock and create a regular sleep routine. Aim to wake up at the same time each day, even at the weekend.

• Have a wind-down routine before going to sleep
Stop doing other activities at least 30 minutes before trying to sleep and do something relaxing instead, e.g. read, have a bath or listen to music. Do not watch TV just before you go to bed as this tends to encourage you to stay up 'just a little bit longer' to see what happens next.

• Only use your bed for sleep

Use your bed only for sleep. Other activities, for example, reading, eating and watching TV, should be done somewhere else. This is because these activities stimulate the brain, which may stop you falling asleep. It is important that you associate bed with sleep and rest, rather than activity.

• If you are not falling asleep in bed get up

Once in bed, if you cannot get to sleep within approximately 20 minutes, it is suggested that you get up, leave the bedroom and do something relaxing. Preferably this should be something un-stimulating, the more boring the better! Return to bed only when you feel drowsy. Use this technique also if you wake in the night and cannot get back to sleep. You may need to get out of bed several times before you eventually get to sleep. The aim is that you begin to associate your bed with sleep rather than stress or activity. Still get up at a regular time the following day, however long you have been asleep during the night.

• Aim to avoid sleeping during the day

It can be easy to sleep in the day if you have not slept well the night before. However, if you are finding it difficult to sleep at night and are falling asleep in the day you will probably make it more difficult for yourself to sleep the following night. This is because you have taken your deep sleep in the day and will therefore need to sleep less at night. When you are tired, aim to avoid daytime sleep. If you want to increase your chances of sleeping for longer at night keep to a regular sleep routine. Go to bed and get up at the same times each day. To reduce catnapping, try to take your nap at the same time each day and for a regular time, e.g. at 1 pm for one hour. (You may need an alarm clock to do this.) Start with an amount that is similar to what your body is trying to take now. Then gradually reduce your daytime sleep, aiming to stop napping in the day altogether if possible.

• Make your sleeping environment conducive to sleep

If your environment is too noisy it can be difficult to sleep. If possible, sleep in the quietest bedroom in the house. If the environment surrounding your bedroom is noisy, close windows and doors to reduce noise, or wear earplugs if you can tolerate this. Some people sleep better with quiet, relaxing music on than listening to background noise. You can experiment to see what works for you. It is also hard to sleep if your room is too light. Make sure you have thick curtains that block out the streetlights and sunlight. Also, make sure lights from the hall or electrical items, like digital clocks, are not shining in your eyes. Make sure you are not too hot or too cold in bed. Also try to make yourself as comfortable as possible before you go to sleep. For example, you may need to take pain killers to reduce pain levels.

• **Eat a snack**

A light supper can help you to sleep. A milky drink, or a banana, contains trytophan, which is thought to convert into serotonin, which is a relaxing, sleep inducing chemical in your nervous system. Some people use up their energy stores very quickly. As your body needs energy overnight for growth and repair, having some slow release carbohydrates, such as wholemeal toast, can help prevent you waking up in the night feeling hungry. Eat your snack around two hours before going to sleep to avoid the process of digestion disturbing your sleep.

• **Avoid stimulants**

Caffeine is in coffee, tea and chocolate. Drinking caffeine prior to going to bed or a lot throughout the day will stimulate the brain and make it harder to sleep. If you have caffeine after 5 pm it can have a negative influence on how you sleep at night. Smoking tobacco results in a release of adrenaline caused by the addictive substance within tobacco, nicotine. Smoking before trying to sleep increases stimulation, at the point when you want to relax and rest. Avoid smoking for an hour before trying to sleep to reduce the impact of the nicotine on your ability to sleep.

• **Avoid alcohol**

As your body breaks down alcohol it impacts on your quality of sleep and can cause you to wake up in the night. If you drink regularly to help you to sleep you could be at risk of becoming dependent on alcohol. It will not help with your sleep difficulties in the long term; in fact it is very likely to make them worse. This is not a problem for many people with CFS/ME as the condition can make it hard to tolerate alcohol.

• Dealing with anxiety

Anxiety is a common cause of sleeping problems. Often you can lie in bed having worrying thoughts go through your head rather than falling asleep. It is common for any concerns or worries to be stronger at night because there is nothing to distract your mind, as there is when you are doing things during the day. Feelings of muscle tension that go with anxious thoughts can make it even harder to fall asleep. People then often start to worry about the fact they cannot sleep, which of course makes sleeping even harder.

The time when you are trying to fall asleep is not the best for thinking about your problems. Write down the problems you think about at night to deal with them in the morning. Have a period of time in the day when you can think about the issues in your life and how to deal with them. It can help to write down ways to resolve your problems. This can be hard as you may need to decide about issues which are important to you, such as relationships and finances. However, the stress that comes with not making a decision is often a lot worse than coping with the consequences of the decision after it has been made.

• Relaxation

When you are asleep your heart rate and breathing rate are slower than when you are awake. If you are stimulated, for example, by worry or excitement, your heart beat and breathing rate are faster. If this is the case when you try to go to sleep, it is very difficult for the body to reduce the heart and breathing level from the high rate of stimulation to the low rate of sleep. Chapter 5 on Stress and Relaxation will give you some ideas on ways of calming your body down before you try to sleep.

• **Medication**

Using medication to help you to sleep may seem like a simple solution to sleep problems, but it can cause new difficulties. While sleeping pills, such as benzodiazepines, can help people fall asleep and decrease anxiety in the short term, these benefits are lost if sedatives are used frequently. This is because if you take medication over a long period of time you become tolerant of the drug, which renders it ineffective. It can also be difficult to stop taking benzodiazepines after taking them for a long time due to the symptoms of anxiety and sleeplessness caused by stopping the medication. In addition, because your body is being artificially put to sleep, the body can actually reduce the amount of sleep hormone that it produces as this is being replaced by the drug. The problem does not, therefore, get any better.

Medication can change the natural sleep cycle, which in turn may negatively affect your quality of sleep. For example, if the medication means you get more R.E.M. sleep than deep sleep, you may dream more but wake up feeling less refreshed. The effect on the sleep cycle varies between different types of medication.

Some people with CFS/ME find that sleeping tablets can add to their fatigue, making them feel 'groggy' in the mornings. It is preferable to use some of the other techniques mentioned in this book to help you to sleep. However, some people with CFS/ME do find medication useful. A doctor may prescribe tricyclic antidepressants to people with persistent lack of sleep. This is at a low dose, so it would be ineffective in treating depression, but at this level is known to help people to sleep without making them feel too 'groggy' in the morning. It can also have a positive effect on pain, which can also help people to sleep better.

Adjusting your sleep pattern

Some people with CFS/ME may be getting enough sleep, but getting their sleep mainly in the day rather than at night - for example, sleeping from 4 am to 1 pm. If this is the case and you want to change it, start by regulating the time you get up. In this example, begin by getting up at 1 pm. (You may need an alarm clock to help you with this.) Then gradually move the time you get up back by half an hour at a time - for example, start getting up at 12.30 p.m. Gradually start to go to bed earlier as you should start to feel tired earlier. Continue this process until you are going to sleep and waking up at the time you want. This process may increase fatigue levels slightly to begin with, but if you stick with it should help you to adjust your sleep pattern with the minimum shock to the system.

Summary

Clinical Practice Guidelines for CFS written by the Australian College of Physicians (2002) states that: 'the aim of sleep management is to establish a regular, normalised sleep-wake pattern'. If you are able to establish a regular sleep routine, it can lead to an improvement in CFS/ME symptoms. It is, therefore, an important issue to address. Do not worry if your sleep routine is not perfect; any improvement can be beneficial. Remember, it is only part of the treatment for CFS/ME and an improvement will be more effective used alongside other measures, such as graded activity.

Sleep checklist

On the next page is a list of the techniques contained in this chapter. The columns on the left allow you to tick off the techniques you have used and record if you have found them helpful. For most people it is a combination of factors that can help to improve their sleep.

Sleep diary

used	helps

Sleeping too much?

used	helps

Gradually reducing amount of sleep

by getting up earlier

Not catnapping

Limiting catnapping

Gradually reducing catnapping

Not sleeping enough

used	helps

Waking up at a regular time

Having a wind down routine

Using your bed only for sleep

Getting up if you are not able to sleep

Avoiding sleeping during the day

Making your environment more

conducive to sleep

Avoiding stimulants

Avoiding alcohol

Dealing with anxiety

Relaxation

Medication

Adjusting your sleep pattern?

used	helps

Gradually moving the sleep pattern

Heather's story

After the onset of CFS/ME, one of the problems I experienced was poor sleep. I found I could not keep going all day and would have to sleep in the afternoons. I was sleeping for between two and three hours everyday. When I woke up after my afternoon sleep I felt awful. The quality of my sleep at night was poor because of muscle pain, headaches and being over tired. I would go to bed, not be able to get to sleep and was often still awake at one o'clock in the morning. I woke up many times throughout the night, often with nightmares. I would sleep lightly for about 30 minutes and then wake suddenly, sweating, and then go into another short, light sleep. This was the pattern of my sleep for a number of years. It took me a long time to get going in the morning and so I got up early to do stretching exercises to ease the muscle stiffness, before taking care of my family before school.

One change that improved my sleep was being prescribed amitriptyline and also understanding what time to take it, to minimise the grogginess I felt in the morning. The medication has improved the quality of my sleep at night thus enabling me to cut out my day time sleep.

I learned that it is helpful to have a routine around sleep and to incorporate that with pacing and grading activity throughout the day, to prevent feeling over tired at bedtime. I kept a sleep diary for a period of time which helped me establish a routine before going to bed. I learned not to watch television, particularly news programmes, before going to bed and to avoid other stimulants, such as demanding discussions and drinking alcohol.

I have established an evening routine starting at nine o'clock, when I have a relaxing bath, and I am in bed before ten o'clock. After taking my medication, I read an easy book until about eleven o'clock, when I go to sleep. I now get up between seven and eight o'clock having had a refreshing sleep and without feeling groggy. Once I was able to sleep through the night, the daytime short sleep could be replaced by a rest if I needed it.

Chapter Four

Diet

Jennifer McIntosh

Introduction

Many people will think about their diet when they experience a problem with their energy levels. Our food is our fuel. It is important to give our bodies the best fuel that we can. There are some advocates for specific diets as a 'cure' for the condition of CFS/ME, but as there are no *evidence-based* dietary remedies, we are not going to look at rigid rules for your diet in this chapter. Instead we will focus on some general principles that many people have found helpful. There are a number of diet factors that do influence the amount of available energy within the human body. For some people making changes in these areas can have a significant impact upon their symptoms. Please use the summary sheet on the next page to note any particular changes that you want to work on.

Summary sheet

Topic	Read	Comments
Diet and CFS/ME		
What should I eat?		
Common problem areas for people with CFS/ME		
Helping energy		
Diet diary		

Diet and CFS/ME

When you are ill it is important to eat a balanced, nutritious diet to give your body the best chance of recovery. People who are experiencing CFS/ME have stated that this is sometimes difficult because they do not have the energy to prepare meals or because their appetite is reduced. This can result in them having an unbalanced diet, which leads to an increase in their fatigue.

Each person is unique, so this book cannot advocate any particular food substance to avoid or to eat more of. Although someone may benefit from avoiding a certain food, others may not. Some people may be prone to certain food intolerances, which become more prominent when they are experiencing

CFS/ME. An inappropriate diet can exacerbate the symptoms of the condition. Many people with CFS/ME also experience, to varying degrees, irritable bowel syndrome (IBS). This may be due to various factors, including the stress of having the condition. What you eat can play a part in this, but beware of making any dramatic changes to your diet - for example, cutting out a certain food group, which will impact on your overall nutritional intake. For more specific dietary advice, please ask your general practitioner for a referral to a dietitian.

In our experience, people find it preferable to stick to a healthy, well balanced diet containing all the components described later in this chapter. Some people choose to investigate alternative diets. If you find a diet that suits you and your health problems, it is reasonable for you to continue with it. However, it is always important to bear in mind that your dietary intake must provide the balanced, nutritional components your body needs.

Research and diets

There have been various recommendations and some published research advocating particular dietary supplements. To date, there has not been any supplement that has consistently been shown in studies to help symptoms significantly. Some supplements are expensive and contain 'mega-doses' of the active ingredient. Large doses of some vitamins, for instance vitamin A and B_6, can be harmful. If you are concerned about your nutritional intake, take a multivitamin and mineral supplement with no more than 100 % of the recommended daily intake. (It can be difficult to know what to take, so please seek professional advice if you are concerned about this.)

A useful question to ask yourself:
• Before we explore more about food, think about what you already know about the six different food groups. What do you think each food group's role is in your health, especially in relation to your CFS/ME?

What should I eat?

In this chapter we are going to look at the elements of a balanced and healthy diet. Although many people are aware of what they *should* be eating, they may not be aware of the importance of each element in relation to their energy and maintaining their body's systems. Often people can be following alternative or exclusion diets without ever having been advised to do so, or without ever having followed a sensible, healthy diet for a period of time. Remember, we do not expect that following a healthy diet will cure your symptoms, but it will help your body to manage the impact that the condition is having upon your health.

Aim to eat a balanced diet, making sure you have the following components in *each* meal:

- Protein
- Carbohydrates
- Fats
- Fruit and vegetables
- Dairy products
- Fluid

Nutrients are best obtained from food rather than supplements or tablets. Remember that if your diet is deficient in one area, supplements may not be effectively absorbed. This is because vitamins and minerals often work in combination with other vitamins, minerals or food components.

Next, we are going to focus on each component of a balanced diet so you can understand what job it does and how to include it in your daily meals.

Protein

Protein can be obtained from a range of different types of foods such as: pulses (beans, peas, lentils), meat, fish, eggs, nuts, quorn, soya alternatives, and baked beans. Protein is essential for growth, repair and the maintenance of every living cell. It is also important in the body's enzyme, hormonal, and immune functions. Many of the B vitamins, iron, magnesium, selenium and zinc are also found in protein-rich foods. Include these in two meals throughout the day. For example, per meal: 1-2 eggs / 75-100 g red meat / 25 g cheese / ½ tin baked beans / 100-150 g white fish / 75-100 g oily fish. A good visual measure is to make a fist with your hand and that indicates your protein portion.

Carbohydrates

Carbohydrates are essential for energy and therefore should make up approximately 50-70 % of your diet everyday. Unrefined complex carbohydrates are also rich in fibre, and B vitamins. There are three types of carbohydrate:

Simple: sugar, glucose, honey, sweets, etc
Starches: white bread, pasta, rice, cornflakes, rice krispies, etc
Complex: wholegrain breakfast cereals, brown rice, wholegrain pasta, wholemeal bread, jacket potatoes, etc

It is important, especially with CFS/ME, that your energy levels remain as constant as possible. You need to remember that the different types of carbohydrate provide energy differently:

- Simple carbohydrates are broken down quickly, providing a quick and short burst of energy. Afterwards, this then leads to a drop in blood sugar levels and a dip in energy levels.
- Starches are broken down slowly, providing a gradual energy release. This sustains your blood sugar level for longer before it then drops.
- Complex carbohydrates are the ideal energy supplier, as they are broken down very slowly. This provides a gradual and even energy release, sustaining energy levels for a longer period. Complex carbohydrates are also high in fibre, which helps regulate your bowels and maintain a sense of fullness.

In CFS/ME it is often suggested that sugar and sugary snacks are excluded, due to some people experiencing a craving for sweet foods when they are fatigued. This can be followed by symptoms similar to reactive hypoglycaemia (a drop in blood sugar). Not everyone will experience these symptoms, but if you do and would still like to include chocolate in your diet, eat it in the evening to avoid energy slumps throughout the day. It helps if you can eat this along with a complex carbohydrate, so that this can start to release energy once the simple carbohydrate has been used up. For example, you could eat a sandwich with wholemeal bread and a chocolate biscuit.

Example meal plan

By incorporating a mixture of carbohydrates into your diet and by eating every two to three hours, you can get the most from your energy levels and help your body work efficiently. Here is an example of foods that will allow you to sustain your energy availability from your diet across the day.

- Breakfast: Bowl of wholegrain cereal, e.g. bran flakes / porridge with semi skimmed milk, or two slices of wholemeal bread spread with margarine/butter and jam.
- Mid-morning: A drink and a banana / two oatcakes / wholemeal scone with jam / cereal bar.
- Lunch: Sandwich made with two slices of wholemeal bread with a filling of your choice and a piece of fruit / yoghurt.
- Mid-afternoon: A drink and two oatcakes / fruit cake / piece of fruit / handful of nuts / cereal bar.
- Evening meal: Wholemeal pasta / brown rice / jacket potato / basmati rice, with fish / meat / eggs / quorn / cheese, and vegetables, plus pudding e.g. stewed fruit and custard / rice pudding / yoghurt.
- Supper: Piece of fruit / 2 biscuits / dried fruit (small handful) / small chocolate bar / bowl of cereal.

Glycaemic index

Another way of ranking carbohydrates is by looking at their glycaemic index (GI). GI is a way of ranking carbohydrate foods based on the rate at which they raise your blood sugar levels. Each food is given a value out of 100.

- Foods that are absorbed quickly are known as *high* glycaemic index. These foods tend to cause a sharp, high rise in blood glucose levels and then a drop.
- Foods that are absorbed slowly are known as *low* glycaemic index foods. These foods produce a gentle rise in blood glucose levels and therefore sustain energy levels for longer.

Ideally aim to eat foods with a low GI as below:

	Low GI	Medium GI	High GI
Drinks	Sugar free drinks	Sports drinks	Glucose drinks
Cereals	Wholegrain cereals e.g. bran flakes		Low fibre cereals e.g. cornflakes
Bread, biscuits, & cake	Heavy-grain bread e.g. granary / multigrain	Fibre-enriched white breads; flapjacks	Brown, wholemeal & white bread; crumpets; water biscuits
Potatoes, rice & pasta	Sweet potatoes, basmati rice, pasta – most types	Boiled & new potatoes; macaroni	Instant, mashed and jacket potato; chips; instant brown and white rice

Fruit & vegetables	Apple, dried apricots, banana, cherries, grapefruit, grapes, kiwi, mango, orange, peach, pear, plum; apple, orange & grapefruit juice; carrots, peas, sweetcorn	Apricots (canned), pineapple, squash, sultanas, raisins	Watermelon, parsnips, pumpkin, swede, broad beans
Pulses / grains	Pulses; pearl barley; buckwheat; bulgar wheat	Cous cous; cornmeal; millet	Tapioca
Snacks	Most chocolate*; popcorn; crisps*; peanuts*	Some chocolate bars* e.g. Mars bars; taco shells	Jelly babies; corn chips
Sugars	Fructose; lactose	Honey; sucrose	Glucose
Dairy	Low-fat ice cream; milk; yoghurt	Full fat ice cream*	

*Foods containing high amounts of fat; aim to eat them only occasionally.

Contradictions to these guidelines include:

- How the food is processed can change the GI value - for example, mashed potato has a higher GI than boiled potatoes.
- If foods are mixed together their GI value will alter - for example, jacket potato (high GI) when mixed with baked beans (low GI) = medium GI.

- Some low GI foods are high in fat*, such as chocolate, so remember to eat it in moderation – e.g. one to two times per week.

Suggestions to improve energy levels:

1. Include one to two portions of low GI foods per day into your diet.
2. Incorporate some complex carbohydrate food into your diet.
3. Aim to eat every two to three hours to help balance your energy levels

> **Useful questions to ask yourself:**
> • Do you think you are eating regularly enough?
> • If not, are there ways of improving your diet to see if your energy levels improve? Start by making one small change - for example, trying a mid-afternoon snack.

Fats

In our diet-conscious world, 'fat' can often be portrayed as our enemy, to be avoided at all cost. However, fats are essential for providing essential fatty acids, which are important in early brain development and for maintaining healthy skin and hair. Fat contains fat soluble vitamins, such as A, E and D, which are important for healthy skin, eyes, hair, etc. Fats are also important for maintenance of heat, protection of vital organs and bringing taste to our food. What we often forget about fats is that they are also a source of energy. Ideally, fats should make up not more than 35% of your total energy requirements.

There are different types of fats; some are more beneficial than others:

Type of fat	Role	Foods
Saturated Ideally aim to reduce	Play a part in increasing total cholesterol in the blood. A high intake therefore may increase the risk of cardiovascular disease	Fats from animals e.g. butter, lard, fatty cuts of meat, cream
Trans fatty acids Aim to reduce	Similar role to saturated fats	Fats that have been dehydrogenated, e.g. pre-cooked vegetable oils, biscuits, cakes, and margarine.
Polyunsaturated Omega 6 To have in moderation, not excess Omega 3 Aim to increase	Key components of phospholipids in membranes, and in the regulation of cholesterol. Two main types: Important in neural development in fetal and early life and anti-inflammatory effect Anti-thrombogenic effect, e.g. protective measure against heart attacks. Plays a very important part in the structure of your brain, retinal, and nervous tissue	Fats from vegetables and plants Sunflower, safflower, corn, groundnut, soya oil, nuts, and margarine Oily fish – mackerel, salmon, sardines, fresh tuna, herring. Flaxseed oil (linseeds)
Monounsaturated Aim to increase	Regarded as one of the most beneficial types of fats as they do not increase cholesterol	Olive, rapeseed and groundnut oil, avocados and nuts

Fruit and vegetables

Fruit and vegetables are particularly high in water soluble vitamins (vitamin C, B_6, folic acid and vitamin K) and minerals (potassium). These are important for a healthy immune system. Vitamins and minerals are best absorbed through food as they interact with each other. Fruit and vegetables are also high in fibre, which is important to regulate your bowels. Aim to eat five or more portions of fruit and vegetables a day.

Guide to food portions for fruit and vegetables	
Vegetables – raw, cooked, frozen, or canned	2-3 tablespoons
Salad	1 dessert bowlful
Grapefruit / avocado pear	½ fruit
Apples, bananas, oranges, etc	1 fruit
Plums, and similar sized fruit	2 fruits
Grapes, cherries and berries	1 cupful or a handful
Fresh fruit salad, stewed or canned fruit	2-3 tablespoons
Dried fruit (raisins, apricots)	½ -1 tablespoon
Fruit juice	1 glass (150 ml)

Remember, frozen fruit and vegetables are just as good as fresh

Dairy products

Dairy products provide the main source of calcium in our diets, which is required for a healthy bone structure. Without adequate calcium you are at risk of developing osteoporosis, which is when the bones become thin and their strength is reduced, making them more likely to break. An ideal calcium intake for adults is between 700 mg to 1000 mg a day.

Good sources of calcium	Points
1 pot (150 g) plain or fruit yogurt / 1/3 pint milk (any type) / 50 g sardines (1/2 tin) in tomato sauce / 50 g tofu	5
30 g cheddar cheese / 30 g edam cheese / 1/3 pint calcium enriched soya milk / large serving of spring greens / spinach, boiled, 130 g	4
1 tbs parmesan cheese / 1 medium cheese scone / ½ small tin pilchards in tomato sauce / 1 scoop dairy ice cream / 3 dried figs / 125 ml (small pot) of calcium-enriched soya yoghurt / 2 slices white or wholemeal bread / 500 ml calcium-fortified mineral water	3
1 pot (100 g) fromage frais / ½ small tin canned salmon / 100 g (small tub) cottage cheese / small bar chocolate / ½ large tin kidney beans	2
1/3 pint soya milk / 3 heaped tsp malted drinks powder / 1 small tin baked beans / 9 Brazil nuts / 8 dried apricot halves / 145 g boiled cabbage	1

Each point = 50 mg calcium; aim for at least 14 points daily

Approximately 1 pint of milk per day, or equivalent, will provide you with an adequate supply of calcium. If for any reason you have reduced your intake of dairy products or have avoided them for a long period of time - for example, one month or more - it is important that you are getting adequate calcium from other sources. There are other foods which are high in calcium and if you would like further advice on this please seek professional support. An important aspect of prevention of osteoporosis is to work on improving your tolerance of weight-bearing activity, such as walking when this is feasible.

Fluid

The human body is around 50-70% water depending on your size and gender. Fluid is lost every day through your kidneys, skin, gut and lungs. It is essential that you replace lost fluids through food and most importantly, drinks. How much you need to drink varies from person to person. However, you need approximately 1.5 litres / 2.5 pints / 8 cups / 5 mugs of fluid per day. The following drinks are ideal: water - bottled or tap; fruit squash can be added (ideally sugar free) - herbal tea, green tea, decaffeinated coffee. Your fluid requirements will increase if your body temperature rises, for instance on a hot summer day, if you have a fever, or with exercise.

Useful questions to ask yourself:
- How much do you think you are drinking?
- Do you need to adjust this?

If you feel you need to drink more, think about what you like and aim to increase your intake by one drink per day or week, depending on what is realistic for you, until you meet your target. Often it helps to carry a small bottle of water or fruit squash with you and take sips throughout the day.

Common problem areas for people with CFS/ME

Caffeine and alcohol

Many people with CFS/ME find caffeine, found in coffee, tea, cola, pro-plus tablets and 'energy' drinks, makes them feel worse and may ultimately drain them of energy. It is best therefore to avoid caffeinated drinks and replace them with decaffeinated varieties, or herbal tea. If this is difficult for you, then aim at least to reduce your intake of caffeinated drinks. Some people find they are unable to drink alcohol as it worsens their symptoms or has a more powerful and unpleasant effect on them. If you do want to drink alcohol, in moderation of course, experiment with various types, as people report that they react differently to different drinks - for example, between beer and spirits.

Weight changes and concerns

It is common in CFS/ME for there to be weight changes, either weight gain or weight loss.

1.   If you gain weight this can be due to a reduction in your activity whilst your appetite remains the same or increases. You may find you are comfort-eating or eating irregularly, as your daily routine has changed. You will find weight loss will be slow. The first aim is to maintain your weight and then to lose 1-2 kg per month. To do this, eat regularly, as we discussed earlier. Reduce the high fat and sugar foods in your diet – for example, crisps, cakes, biscuits, sugary drinks and chocolate. Increase your intake of vegetables and fruit and incorporate low glycaemic foods into your diet.

2.   It is common to lose weight if you are suffering from nausea, your appetite has reduced or you forget meals due to poor concentration and memory problems. Aim to eat every two to three hours and incorporate high energy foods such as milkshakes, nuts, crackers, cheese, cake and easy meals into your diet. Avoid drinking at meal times, so you do not fill up on fluids. Instead sip drinks

in between your meals. If you have problems with nausea eat drier foods - for example, crackers and foods that do not have a strong smell. Foods containing ginger can also help.

Food allergy and intolerance

Food allergy and food intolerance often seem to be linked in the same sentence. However they are different problems.

A **food allergy** is an immediate reaction, sometimes severe, by the body to a protein found in a particular food, for example shellfish. In response, our bodies produce *IgE antibodies*, which then cause the reaction. This usually occurs immediately after eating the food. This also means that there are some clear diagnostic tests for allergies - for example, allergen specific IgE blood tests and skin prick tests. These can be carried out through your GP.

Food intolerance is an adverse reaction to a food which occurs when our bodies have an inability to digest that food successfully. This can often manifest as bowel symptoms. There is currently not enough clinical evidence to show that avoiding a particular food will reduce fatigue, improve concentration, or reduce muscle pain. Also, food intolerance means you can still tolerate that food(s) in small amounts. This means you do not need to avoid it completely, as this can increase problems tolerating that food in the longer term. Currently there are no diagnostic tests for food intolerances, although there are many companies that claim that they are able to do this. If you suspect you have a food intolerance, we suggest you keep a food and symptom diary for two weeks, to monitor if there is a link between your symptoms and your diet.

If you have a diagnosis of food allergy or suspect a food intolerance, ask to be referred to a dietitian to discuss this further. This is to ensure that you do not start excluding the suspected food from your diet if this might affect your nutritional balance. For example, excluding dairy products will reduce your calcium intake unless you replace them with an appropriate substitute.

Helping energy

Healthy eating need not take more effort than before!

How you prepare your food can also reduce your energy. Consider your movements around the kitchen and the way you have things laid out. How can you make it easier for yourself? Avoid undertaking exhausting, complex tasks all at once. Think creatively about ways in which you can break down the task into manageable parts that can be spread out over time. For example, it may help to peel vegetables in the morning and get out ingredients earlier than you would usually. Include rest periods in your planning and find a pace which suits you.

Be aware of when you eat

We have found that people with CFS/ME benefit from eating small amounts on a regular basis - for example, dividing up the larger meals into smaller amounts and eating every two hours. This is sometimes called 'grazing'. This ensures that your body is getting a constant supply of energy throughout the day and does not have to digest large meals.

Ensure you have a short rest period (around 20 minutes) or only attempt low-grade activity after eating, to aid digestion. In addition, do not eat for around two hours before you go to bed. Eating just before going to bed can disturb your sleep patterns, leading to lower energy levels.

Other factors to consider in your diet

Different diets can involve lengthy, energy sapping shopping trips in order to find the right products. If this is so, think of ways to simplify the journey or have the ingredients delivered. Make sure that the benefits outweigh the disadvantages, in terms of energy spent. Some people find it easy to cook in bulk as they are doing each individual task anyway. Freeze the excess for a day when you have less energy available to cook.

Remember

The most important thing is to eat and drink regularly and have a balanced diet. If you are not eating regularly your body will not have the energy it needs and this will increase your fatigue levels.

Finally, there is an eating diary included in this chapter, which you can use to record what, how often and how much you are eating and drinking; you can use your own method of doing this. Think about this and what changes to your diet might be helpful for you to increase your energy supplies. If you have specific problems with your digestive system, food intolerances or with your weight, then you may benefit from consulting a registered dietitian to look at your individual requirements.

Useful resources

- Thomas B, Bishop J (2007) *Manual of Dietetic Practice* 4th edition. Oxford: Blackwell Publishing
- Collins, C (Dec 2007) *Osteoporosis Food Facts Sheet.* British Dietetic Association

Diet diary

For the next 5-7 days write down everything you are eating and drinking during that day. If possible aim to keep the diary as you go along, as it can be hard to remember details at the end of the day. Next, think about what you can change to improve your diet.

Day:

Time and place	Food eaten	Quantity
For example, were you at home at the table or in front of TV or out at a friend's	Be specific - for example, name the brand of the product	For example, how many slices of bread or size of potato

Georgina's story

I have always had an interest in diet and nutrition. After developing CFS/ME, I struggled to incorporate what I already knew about healthy eating into my life, so that it did not aggravate my irritable bowel syndrome (IBS), was low fat and met my needs in terms of budget and family life.

With regard to my IBS, I learned that avoiding onions and hard-skinned fruits and vegetables is beneficial. I also learned to avoid caffeine, which I found makes me tired almost immediately after consuming it. I found coffee affects my IBS symptoms and tea affects my energy levels. I now have decaffeinated drinks. I also found that alcohol increases my fatigue so I avoid alcohol completely.

I have noticed that my appetite has increased since having CFS/ME and so one of my concerns is weight gain. I was confused about whether to eat to keep my energy levels up or not to eat so much so as to maintain my weight. I have been advised to eat small portions regularly so that I keep my blood sugar constant. I used to snack on fatty and sugary foods, which I knew were not good for me. Now I make sure that I eat something every two to three hours and that I choose a healthy option. I find plain chocolate is great for giving me a boost when I feel I need it. I have discovered that eating a large meal does increase my fatigue. I have also found that I need to eat or drink something so that I can rest beneficially.

I kept a food diary for a week so that I could monitor what I ate and how it affected my fatigue. I noticed that when I was particularly fatigued, I had cravings for sugary foods. I still notice that there are times when I do not feel full or satisfied even when I have eaten.

One thing I have learned is to lower my expectations about myself. I wanted to provide a nutritious meal for my family everyday. I now realise that sometimes I do not have enough energy to cook and that I am doing the best I can. I prepare vegetables, and then freeze them for times when I am feeling too poorly to cook from scratch. It means I always have something in the freezer that I can stir fry or boil, so I know my family are getting the nutrition they need. I often eat my main meal of the day at lunchtime and then prepare something for my children in the evening. Also, I always ensure I have food in my freezer and cupboards that I can microwave quickly and easily if I need to.

I am getting better at planning and organising myself. When I am writing my shopping list I make sure I check what I have in the cupboards, so that I can plan my meals around what I have available. I conserve my energy by shopping online and having the food delivered, or I ask someone to help me with carrying and unloading my bags if possible. I plan simple meals, which also take into account my budget. I buy 'two for one' offers at the supermarket and look at the shelves where food is discounted when it is due to go out of date. Sometimes I make enough food to last for two meals so that I only have to cook once in two days.

One thing which I have benefited from is carrying a carton of juice and a snack bar with me when I am out. I always have something to eat and drink to give my energy levels a boost if I need to.

Chapter Five

Stress and Relaxation

Katie Lorentz

Introduction

Stress is a normal and necessary part of everyday life. It helps you to do the things that you need to do. However, sometimes the level of stress you feel can make it harder to get on with your life. Having CFS/ME can often make your life more stressful. In addition, stress can also have a direct impact upon your symptoms of CFS/ME.

This chapter is intended to help you to reflect upon what is meant by stress and how you respond to it. Having more understanding about the effects of stress on your body, mind and actions can help you to think about different ways that you can respond to stress in your life. This will therefore help you in the management of your energy and limiting the impact of stress on your symptoms.

Summary sheet

Topic	Read	Comments
What is stress?		
The evolution of your body's response to demand		
How does this affect you?		
The stress-response biological pathway		
Assess how you respond to stress		
Managing stress		
Stress and your body - relaxation		
Stress and your mind		
Stress and your actions		
Summary		

What is stress?

Here are the thoughts of some people who have CFS/ME about the stress that they experience:

'I keep meaning to get a little time for myself but I never manage to. Someone always asks me to help out and I never have the heart to say no and I end up feeling really tired and irritable.'

'I see all the things piling up that I feel I should be doing. I worry that I will never catch up. In the past I would be able to do every-thing with no trouble.'

'I can't cope with being around lots of people any more, so I avoid the supermarket. I feel less fatigued if I go when no one else is around.'

Stress is a normal part of everyday life. Everyone experiences stress to some extent, and in some situations it actually enhances performance - for example, in an exam or interview. However, stress can start to cause problems in situations where demand is perceived to outweigh resources - for example, when the demands on your energy exceed your supply of energy. Remember the model of supply and demand you were introduced to in Chapter 1, see the diagram below. As this is in the nature of having CFS/ME, then experiencing stress caused by the condition can be a common issue.

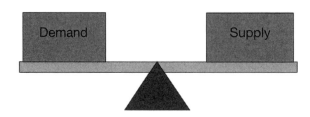

The importance of balancing demand and supply.

It is very common to be a little anxious or stressed in some everyday situations and that can help you to get things done. Sometimes you may feel very highly stressed about things you believe are important, but other people do not feel the same. This can lead you to feel embarrassed and not wanting to talk about how you feel. It then makes it more likely that you will get 'worked up' and this can result in avoiding stressful situations altogether.

The evolution of your body's response to demand

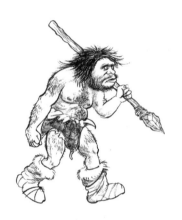

To understand more about how our bodies generate energy in response to demand or threat, we need to go back to the time when our ancestors were hunter/gatherers. To help us to explain this we are going to use the story of 'Fred' the caveman.

In Fred's world everything is about survival and the key to survival is to be able to hunt food, build shelter and fight off predators – all of which require energy. Resources, such as food, are scarce, so Fred does not want to produce high levels of energy all of the time. Only at the times he really needs it. The body has had to evolve systems for varying the amount of energy it produces in response to the situation.

The first stage is that his brain needs to recognise what is a threat or a demand. So when his thinking processes identify this, it then triggers a response in his central nervous system and the release of certain hormones. These activate the required changes in his body.

The first significant change is the increase in the activity of his body's 'engine' – namely, his heart and lungs to get more oxygen, and from this to get energy into his body. The body also targets where it wants the increase in energy to go. In Fred's world he needs to hunt or fight. This requires the large muscle groups in his body, like his arms and legs, to work harder. Therefore, more blood is sent to the muscles that are needed for this. In addition, the internal tension in each muscle cell, which is shaped like a coil, is increased to hold that energy ready to be released.

There are two major body systems that Fred does not need at this time, so blood is diverted away from those organs. The digestive system, which takes a lot of blood flow and energy to operate, is put on standby. The reproductive system is also affected, as this is also not needed at this time!

He needs to make quick decisions, so more blood is sent to his brain and the electrical activity in his brain is speeded up. More information is taken in through his senses to enable Fred to be more vigilant to what is happening around him.

In this way Fred improves his performance and is more likely to survive in a fight. When the threat has passed, he can then go back to his cave and relax. At this time the response switches into its opposite mode, so that he can relax and conserve energy for when it will be needed again.

How does this affect you?

This system still works very effectively and helps you in threatening, or particularly demanding, situations to produce the extra energy that you need. These physiological changes are often known as the *fight or flight* response or stress response. However, the world has changed. Most of the things that are a demand on you now are not things you need physically to fight or to run away from. With CFS/ME it is things like health concerns, work, money and family that are demands, and they do not usually require a short-term physical reaction. However, the body's system works the same as it has always done. Let us think about what happens if it gets switched on and not switched back off again!

When you start to think about a threat or demand, adrenaline is released. This increases your breathing, heart rate and blood pressure. The muscle fibres recoil like springs, ready to release their energy. If they are not used - for example, in the physical action of fighting or running away - they remain tense, and begin to hurt and shake.

Blood is diverted from your digestive system, causing problems such as heartburn, constipation and diarrhoea. Salivation is decreased, causing a dry mouth. Your thoughts also speed up. As you are focused on the demand you are dealing with, this then releases more adrenaline to help you to do this, thus keeping the system switched on. This creates a vicious cycle. In addition, as the production of energy creates heat, your temperature increases, and you may begin to sweat or blush.

All of these physical changes, which at times may feel very unpleasant, are part of your body's natural responses. They were designed to help human beings, like Fred, survive. However, although the system is designed to help you, sometimes it can become a problem. If due to dealing with a number of demands at once, which is often the case in CFS/ME, you start to experience some of these reactions, such as muscle pain, headaches, shortness of breath, etc, you may not realise that you could be experiencing the legacy of your ancestors. You may become concerned as to why you are feeling so physically ill and not realise the impact that this reaction is now having upon your health and specifically upon your CFS/ME symptoms.

The stress-response biological pathway

Some people find it helpful to know more about the biological processes that occur in the body during this reaction. If this does not interest you, move on to the next section. For those who think they will find it helpful, here is a basic explanation of some of the biological mechanisms involved in this response.

There are two parts to the autonomic nervous system – **sympathetic** and **parasympathetic** – which work in opposition to each other. This means they cannot work at the same time. The response described in Fred is the sympathetic response. This helps us to perform, be active and meet the demands of life.

In comparison, the parasympathetic response helps our bodies to maintain themselves over the longer term, such as getting nutrients and energy from food, handling repairs and growth of cells, and fighting infection. Many

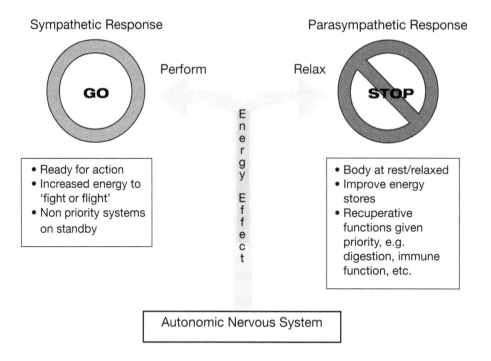

people assume that these functions of the parasympathetic nervous system happen automatically while they are asleep. However, they only occur if you are *relaxed* while you are sleeping. It is possible to sleep and still have sympathetic responses occurring- for example, if your brain is still working hard to make sense of your illness, or if you are constantly moving due to pain or having bad dreams, etc. So sometimes the parasympathic system may not be getting sufficient chance to do its work, because the sympathetic system is dominating.

Assess how you respond to stress

You may experience a range of different physiological and emotional responses to stress. An important step in managing this for you to become more aware of your own body and mind.

Task

Listed below are some of the common signs of stress. Tick the signs that you recognise in yourself. These may be the signs that you have always experienced in response to stress or you may have found that these have changed since experiencing CFS/ME.

Physical signs	Tick		Tick
Headaches		Breathlessness	
Muscle tension or pain		Palpitations	
Stomach problems		Dry mouth	
Sweating		Tingling in the body	
Feeling dizzy		Sexual problems	
Bowel or bladder problems			

Emotional signs	Tick		Tick
Irritability		Apathy	
Anxiety and tension		Low self-esteem	
Low mood			

Behavioural signs	Tick		Tick
Losing temper more easily		Being unreasonable	
Increased drinking/smoking		Being forgetful/distracted	
Changes in eating habits		Getting more clumsy	
Withdrawing from usual activity		Rushing around	

Obviously many of these signs can also be caused by high levels of fatigue. So it can become difficult for you to differentiate between when these symptoms are related to your CFS/ME and when they are related to dealing with all the demands that you are trying to cope with. In some ways it does not matter, because the things that can be helpful in dealing with stress will also benefit the physiological symptoms of your condition. Remember, the parasympathetic nervous system is responsible for aiding digestion, supporting the function of your immune system, healing and regeneration of the body, as well as energy conservation. So, helping yourself to switch from the sympathetic response (that is associated with 'doing' and demand) to the parasympathetic response (that is associated with 'relaxing') will help the natural healing and essential maintenance mechanisms in your body to work.

Managing stress

Managing your stress more effectively not only means that you will reduce the risk of other health problems such as heart disease, high blood pressure, depression and stomach ulcers, but also reduce the energy used by the stress response, leaving energy for other things. This follows the theory of the energy bank discussed in chapter one, whereby you are trying to reduce the things that take energy away from you and increase the things that give you energy.

The first step in managing stress more effectively is to understand what happens when you are stressed and why. The second is to identify the triggers of your stress in your everyday life, and how you currently respond to these. The third is to begin to learn new ways of responding to potentially stressful situations.

Task

Take a moment to assess how you are feeling. Consider your physical and emotional state. This is not always easy to do, and many of us are not aware of how this can change throughout any one day. Check in with yourself on a regular basis, and note how you are feeling. Become accustomed to what clues your body gives you. What are the warning signs that you are becoming stressed, tense or worried?

There are three main areas – physical, thoughts and behaviour - through which stress can be targeted, as illustrated in the diagram opposite. The next sections will look at each of these areas in turn to help you to think about ways to reduce stress.

Stress and your body – relaxation

In chapter two, we considered the benefits of relaxation in the context of improving the quality of your rest. As being 'relaxed' is a key strategy in recovery from CFS/ME and because it goes beyond just the state of resting, we are going to explore this further. Relaxation is the opposite of stress, or high arousal. In a relaxed state you can feel calm and confident, with reduced tension in your body and mind. This is when you are in the parasympathetic response. There are different levels of feeling relaxed, in the same way as you will experience different

Changes in how your body feels

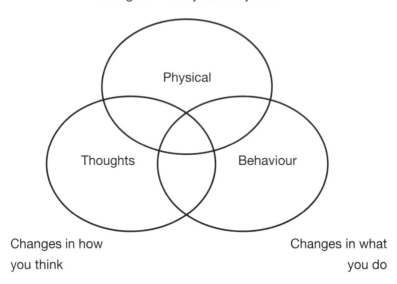

Changes in how
you think

Changes in what
you do

levels of stress. Sometimes this may be at a deep level - for example, when you are in a deep sleep. However, it is possible to experience a degree of relaxation whilst doing an activity - for example, doing something you enjoy with no pressures or distractions.

Why is relaxation helpful?

- When you are stressed, the muscles in your body are tense. If this state is prolonged, this can cause uncomfortable aches and pains such as headache, backache and other muscular pains. By relaxing, you are allowing the muscles to be tension free. Relaxation is commonly used within pain management programmes, and it can be a good strategy for reducing the effects of the muscular pain experienced in CFS/ME.
- People who are tense often feel tired. Holding a tense position uses more energy than being in a relaxed one. By relaxing properly you conserve energy, because your muscles are not working as hard and this is beneficial for the overall management of your condition.

- Being tense requires an increase in blood volume to the 'fight or flight' muscles, such as in the legs and arms, at the expense of the stomach and other systems not required for this response. This means that the digestive system slows down, so digestive problems such as irritable bowel syndrome (IBS) or indigestion can follow. By relaxing you are able to improve your digestion, and minimise stomach problems, which can also be an issue for people with CFS/ME.
- Tension can lead to difficulties getting comfortable and therefore getting to sleep at night. Relaxation can help aid restful sleep.
- Research has shown a link between high stress levels and poor immune system function, as well as being a cause of heart related conditions. Relaxation can help to boost the immune system, and support recovery in CFS/ME.

Relaxation is something that everybody can benefit from. However, for people with CFS/ME it is especially important. This is because of the energy that relaxation conserves. It is also important as having CFS/ME can limit the other ways you could physically manage your stress, such as taking more exercise.

Relaxation guidelines

Relaxation is a skill, which has to be learned through practice. There are a variety of specific techniques that you can learn to help you with relaxation. These include simple breathing exercises (see page 106), meditation, learning how to tense and relax different muscles (which can be called progressive muscular technique) and using your imagination to take you to somewhere where you can feel relaxed (which can be called guided fantasy). There are usually books and CDs available at local stores or through the internet that can help you to learn different techniques to find which suits you or, if you are able to manage it, local classes may be available.

Start by using relaxation strategies in less stressful situations, such as during a quiet time in the day or before going to sleep, then extend your practice to more stressful situations. Then, eventually, implement the techniques in everyday life. It can also be difficult to start practising these techniques when your fatigue level is at its highest, due to the impact that this has upon your concentration. Therefore, start by using them on the days when you feel able to and then increase the number of times that you do so. Awareness is the key. Through using relaxation techniques, you will begin to recognise your body and mind's levels of relaxation and any existing tension. The aim is to gain more control over the level of tension, so that you can reduce it and become more relaxed.

We recommend that you leave about 30 minutes between eating and your relaxation practice, as a full stomach can make relaxation more difficult. Aim to stay awake during your relaxation practice if you are able to, so that you can consciously recognise and experience the state of relaxation. However, you can choose to use a relaxation CD to help you with getting to sleep if you have difficulty sleeping.

Immediately following your practice, take your time coming out of the state of deep relaxation and have a drink of water. This helps with returning you to a more alert state again, and gives you time for planning what you might want to do next. Once you have mastered any of the relaxation techniques, you can use them whenever you experience tension or anxiety, or as part of your rest routine. It is best used as a preventative measure, not in a reactive manner. The key is to keep practising, and make these techniques part of your life.

Useful questions to ask yourself:
If you are not someone who has had time for relaxation, it can feel difficult at the beginning. Take it one step at a time. Ask yourself:
- When do you feel most relaxed?
- What are you doing?
- Who are you with?
- What time of day is it?

Leisure activities, such as watching TV, reading or socialising, are often mistaken for relaxation. These things are activities, which *may* or *may not* be relaxing. You may find that they enable you to feel more relaxed than doing other types of activities, or even than sitting doing nothing. This is still a good start. Plan your day so that you do more relaxing activities on a regular basis. However, it must not stop there. Take the level of relaxation that you can achieve during these times and work on improving on it. A good way to start is by carrying out simple breathing exercises. Extend the time you do this for and build it into good quality relaxation. You may find the following technique helpful. Attempt to practise it regularly throughout the day. The more you practise, the better you get and the more effectively the technique works.

Task: Abdominal breathing technique

It is very difficult to breathe properly when tense or in a high demand situation. See what happens when you hold your stomach in, tensing your muscles, and then try to take a deep breath.
To help your breathing follow these steps:

- Breathe out through your mouth and let your shoulders drop right down.
- Concentrate on your stomach and let the muscles of your stomach completely relax; your stomach should be rounded.
- Take a slow breath in through your nose and let your stomach expand outwards with the in-breath.
- Hold the breath for two or three seconds with your stomach remaining as relaxed as possible.
- Now, let the breath go, breathing out through your mouth. Breathe out all the air in your lungs.
- Let your stomach fall gently back down with your out-breath.

Repeat this technique frequently, breathing normally after every three abdominal breaths you take.

Are you doing it correctly?

It is very easy to take a deep breath in, but this can often make your muscles feel tenser if you are not doing it in the correct way. It can also make you feel dizzy. Therefore, the most important element of this breathing technique is concentrating on letting your stomach relax. This allows your diaphragm to drop down into your abdomen and therefore allow your chest to expand fully.

To test you are doing the technique correctly, place a hand on your stomach just below your ribs or over your navel. This hand should gently rise when you breathe in and fall as you breathe out.

Stress and your mind

Your body and mind are not separate; they are part of the same system. This is why your thoughts and feelings influence how you feel physically and vice versa. Think about what happens when you watch a scary horror film. Your body can react as if it is actually facing the danger shown on screen. Sometimes the threat is in what you are thinking - for example, what you have forgotten to do, or not had the energy to do, or bills that are due; worrying about a loved one's safety; or pondering over how your condition is going to affect your future. In addition, the physical response to stress explored earlier can easily be misinterpreted as signs of a worsening of your CFS/ME. It can then increase your worry about your health, which will in turn increase your stress response and, as a consequence, increase the intensity of the symptoms you are experiencing. This creates a vicious cycle. However, you will not always be aware of the thoughts that you are experiencing. An important part of managing stress is becoming more aware of your thoughts, and the response that they may be triggering. The next chapter will look at thoughts in more detail and how to deal with these. In this chapter we will focus on one strategy that can be helpful: diverting your thoughts.

Distraction

Distraction can be a useful tool in some circumstances. This involves focusing your mind on something other than what is worrying you. For example, focusing on watching a film may distract you from thinking about all the things you feel you ought to be doing but feel too fatigued to do. There are countless other activities than can be used as distraction. In fact, anything that you have to concentrate on will keep the worries from your mind. However, beware, it is only advisable to use this technique for situations or demands that you can do nothing to change. Distraction does not solve a problem or help to change a situation. If it is an ongoing issue, such as worrying about your health, it is likely that as soon as you try to relax or go to sleep, the worrying thoughts will come back into your mind. In addition, it is important to remember that distraction uses energy. Make sure that the activity that you are using for the purpose of distraction is within your baseline level of energy. Otherwise, it may stop you doing something more important later on.

> **Useful questions to ask yourself:**
> Think about when you use distraction (we all do at some time or other).
> - What activities or mental exercises work well for you?
> - When do you use them, and for how long?
> - Do they encroach into your rest time, or cause you to go beyond your baseline?

Sometimes people find that although distraction activities can push them beyond their baseline level, this is still better than sitting and worrying, and sometimes uses less energy too. If this is the case, think about the least demanding activities that you could use. Over time, it may be more helpful to develop a problem-solving approach, and to rely less on distraction.

Task

- Write down the issue or situation that is bothering you. (This can feel awkward at first, but it means you can focus on one thing at a time, and refer to it at a later date when needed).

- Next, write down possible options, actions or solutions for that situation – however unrealistic or undesirable they may seem. (This is to encourage creative thinking and to explore all potential options.)

- Pick the one that you prefer or is most realistic within your current level of symptoms. Write down a plan to carry out the action required. (Remember that this may have to be graded – one step at a time.)

• You can repeat this process as many times as is necessary. You may come up with different options each time you do it.

• If you are still prone to worrying about the situation, set yourself 'worry' and 'non-worry' times during the day. Write down when you will have your 'worry' time.

Stress and your actions

You can reduce the impact of your stress response by altering some of the things that you do. Sometimes people can find certain situations so stressful that they avoid them, either partially or completely. Everyone does this to a certain extent, whether it is paying a bill, telling someone something that they may not wish to hear, washing up, or doing something that you are afraid of. In the short term this can reduce the level of stress experienced. However, some things cannot be avoided, and the longer you put them off for, the worse they can seem to get. Making a plan of how you are going to deal with a certain situation can be helpful. Bear in mind the principles of energy management in relation to your current baseline.

People with CFS/ME often put off dealing with a situation they know will be stressful for them until a day when they feel their energy levels are high enough for them to cope. This may work for you. However, delaying addressing the situation may create more stress, because it could cause other problems as a result, or you may worry that it has not been done. One solution is to break the task down and do one thing towards managing the situation that is within your energy levels, even if you cannot do the whole task.

Lifestyle can have a big impact on your stress levels. Making sure you eat a sensible diet and have regular sleep patterns gives your body greater resources to cope with stress. It is also helpful to begin to recognise the things that put you under pressure or increase the amount of stress that you experience.

> **Useful questions to ask yourself:**
> Think about a situation that is currently causing you some stress.
>
> • How can you begin to reduce the demand of this situation, or the amount of energy that you allow yourself to give over to it?
> • Can you change what you do in response to the situation?

Summary

We hope that you have found the information in this chapter useful, and have experimented with different strategies for managing your stress. If you feel that stress still presents a problem in managing your condition, there are lots of approaches that might help you. These include things such as meditation, massage, and counselling. If you find that stress significantly affects your CFS/ME symptoms and, having tried self-help strategies, you are still struggling to cope with this, please remember that you can speak to a health professional for further advice. Remember too that some of these approaches take time to learn and to experience the benefit of. Be patient, and if you really feel that something is not working, use a different approach. Keep going until you find a strategy that works for you. Remember that any reduction in stress can lead to a reduction in fatigue.

Useful resources

- Gleitman H, Fridlund A, Reisberg D (2004) *Psychology*, 6th edition. New York: Norton
- Looker T, Gregson O (2003) *Managing Stress*. London: Hodder Headline

Jill's story

I have been severely affected by CFS/ME for the past 11 years. I was a teacher and led a busy life, both professionally and socially. At the start of the illness I experienced stress because, as my health deteriorated, I felt guilty for letting people down and not being able to keep to arrangements I had made. I continued to push myself and was determined not to be off work with ill health. In time, I was forced to reduce my hours to part-time and eventually to change to supply teaching. I told myself that I would do a certain number of hours per week, and yet when someone rang to ask if I could work over and above those hours, I found myself saying yes and so putting increased pressure on myself. In addition, I found supply teaching stressful because I only knew which school I was going to with short notice.

I found it difficult to switch my mind off and I was experiencing frequent headaches. I was not sleeping well and a lot of the time I felt too ill to sleep. I was in pain, which was exacerbated by the stress and tension I was feeling. On the outside I appeared calm and inside I was experiencing frustration and anger. When someone asked me how I was feeling I would tell them I was 'OK', and they would think I was being positive towards being ill. Inside I was feeling incredibly low and desperate about what was happening in my life.

I owned my own home and enjoyed spending time outside. I liked walking and being with people. Over time all the things I had loved to do became less and less possible and my self-esteem was eroded. I became housebound and was more, and more, reliant on other people. My health deteriorated to the point where I did not have the strength to push up the sash windows or open a tin of cat food. I felt suicidal and after reaching my lowest point, I spent time at a respite centre. There I met Sue, whom I now live with and who has cared for me for the past eight years.

Over the years I have received a huge amount of support, and with regard to stress, I have learned techniques for managing it. Breathing exercises have been helpful and I now do some of these every morning. I concentrate on the out-breath and on breathing deeper and slower. I also meditate. Since starting to practise both meditation and the breathing exercises, I have been able to see the benefits I have got, in terms of feeling calmer and not being so emotional about things. In the past, a lot of my energy was being used on emotions. Breathing and meditation techniques have helped me not to get sucked into my emotions so often. That means I do not worry as much now if someone says something which in the past I would have taken personally or as being a criticism. I am not as worried that I may have said something to someone and inadvertently upset them. I am not using as much energy on my negative emotions, so I feel less drained and generally happier.

I can now see that much of the stress I used to feel I put on myself. Being severely ill brought with it stress because I could not go out of the house. Also, I experienced stress due to worries - for example, about needing carers who came three times a day. The expectations I put on myself cause me to feel stress. I can see how I can set myself up to feel stressed by setting my expectations too high. I have begun to experience the benefits of pleasure without feeling guilty about enjoying myself.

My appetite has improved as a result of my mood improving and because I do not feel as upset so often. I am now enjoying food and I do not get as worried about what I am eating and how it might affect my health. In the past I had restricted my diet because I was suffering from irritable bowel syndrome (IBS) and was very concerned about what I ate.

Realising that I can laugh at myself has been significant in helping my health to improve. When I have thoughts which I know are unrealistic, I can recognise them more easily now and see the humour in them. I am feeling less tense and, therefore, I am not experiencing the degrees of pain I once did. Sometimes I put on a silly hat, look in the mirror and laugh at myself!

I recently went away overnight, which was a huge step for me. In the past I would have been extremely fearful of taking such a step. This time I actually found myself looking forward to it. The trip was to Ilkley, only six miles from where I live. In the past I would have thought that too insignificant to even bother aiming for. By setting realistic expectations of myself, I was able to look forward to this holiday and enjoy being away whilst I was there. I had previously told myself that a holiday would be when I was well enough to go to Ireland. It means I can now enjoy living in the moment.

Working on building my self-confidence has meant I feel more in control and less affected by other people and events. That means I feel less stressed and I have fewer headaches. People have also commented that my voice sounds stronger and my face looks more relaxed. Nowadays, I can more easily recognise when I am feeling stressed and I tell myself that feelings and thoughts come and go. In the past I could not change my feelings and thoughts. I know that my thoughts influence my moods. When I am feeling stressed, I work on bringing to mind happy memories and images. In the past I struggled to admit that I was feeling anxious. Now that I can admit those feelings to myself and not see them as being a weakness, I do not feel as fearful of feeling anxious.

When I find my thoughts are racing, I work on focusing on what I am doing, which in turn slows my thoughts down. I accept that at times I am not able to relax completely and that relaxation is a gradual process which I cannot force. It is still beneficial to concentrate on my breathing, even if I am not able to relax fully immediately.

Chapter Six

Thoughts and Feelings

Suzanne Moore and Clare Redmond

Introduction

The effects of living with CFS/ME can cause changes in your life which may be stressful and distressing. In any illness, the way we *think* about our symptoms and the impact they have can affect how we feel about them and how we manage them. For example, if a person with diabetes thinks, 'There is nothing I can do to control my illness', then they may not do things that are helpful for this condition - for example, watching their diet, monitoring their blood sugar, taking their insulin and exercising. On the other hand, if they think, 'I do have some control here; there are many things that I can do to manage my diabetes', then they are more likely to do things that *would* help.

These ideas can also be used in managing other health problems, like CFS/ME. There may be times when you find it difficult to be positive - for example, during a relapse. It can be hard adjusting your life, especially if you have had to restrict the things that you do everyday. At times you may feel frustrated, demoralised or worried about your health and the problems it causes.

These responses are understandable and reasonable. It is normal to experience a number of strong emotions. Adjusting to any chronic illness or physical condition requires change that can affect everything about you. This chapter focuses on how to cope with this aspect of having CFS/ME.

Summary sheet

Topic	Read	Comments
Dealing with change and loss		
Managing your thoughts and feelings		
How do your thoughts connect with what is happening to you?		
How do your thoughts connect with your feelings?		
How do your thoughts connect with your physical reactions?		
How do your thoughts connect with how you behave?		
When is a thought unhelpful?		
How to challenge your thoughts		
Looking for evidence		
Testing things out		
What to do next		

Managing your mood		
Managing anxiety		
Summary		

Dealing with change and loss

Having to cope with change and loss is a major issue for many people facing on-going health problems. With CFS/ME you may experience a number of losses, such as work or family roles, even feeling like you are not the same person anymore. It is completely natural to experience many different emotions in response to this. You may feel shock and disbelief at the changes happening in your life. Denial is common. You may reassure yourself that things are alright and believe that this is not really happening. Frustration, anger and anxiety are typical emotions that come with change. There can be a tendency to blame others, such as doctors, or to have a sense of not being in control. Low mood can also be a normal emotion in response to loss. You may have experimented with new ways of doing things, building into your life ways to manage your CFS/ME. This can give you a feeling of hope. It is common to go back and forth through all these different emotions.

We recognise that for some people the typical feelings of sadness and worry may persist and develop into a depressive or anxiety disorder. If this is the case for you then the advice at the end of this chapter may help. You will find information on the signs and symptoms of anxiety and depression, as well as on the types of support and treatment available. It is useful to bear in mind that there is sometimes confusion about the differences between depression and CFS/ME. It is important to be clear that these are two separate conditions, but they can exist at the same time in the same person.

Managing your thoughts and feelings

You may recall from the last chapter, on 'Stress and Relaxation', that your thoughts and feelings (emotions) influence how you feel physically. This chapter will go on to show you the links between how you think, how your feel and how you act. It will introduce you to some of the ways to find and challenge any thoughts that may be unhelpful to how you manage your CFS/ ME. The techniques are largely based on the principles of cognitive behavioural therapy (CBT).

The cognitive behavioural model

The basis of CBT is that how you interpret a particular situation (present, past or future) will influence how you feel and behave. The CBT model covers four connected areas: thoughts, feelings, behaviour and physical changes. There is a fifth area which takes into account the situation that you are currently thinking about. Each area will have an effect on each of the others. For example, whilst you are reading this you may automatically think, 'This is too hard to follow', and so feel despondent and put the book down. On the other hand you may have a different thought, such as, 'This seems a bit complicated; I had better take my time to read it', and as a result, give yourself more time to do so. The effect of this thought does not create the same emotions and reaction as the first.

So, how you think about a problem can affect how you feel emotionally and also how you behave as a result. It can also have an effect on your physical symptoms. A common example would be thinking about all the jobs you think that you *should* be doing, which makes you feel *guilty*, so you become *more active* because of this, and you experience *more fatigue* as a result. The following describes the four areas.

Thoughts

There are three different levels of thought. These levels are commonly referred to as **automatic thoughts**, **assumptions/rules** and **beliefs**. Assumptions and core beliefs are often developed in childhood. This chapter focuses on automatic thoughts.

- **Automatic thoughts** as the name implies are automatic; they pop into your mind spontaneously throughout the day. Often these thoughts are rapid and brief. Most of the time you have no awareness of them. Sometimes the automatic thoughts can be in the form of images or memories.

- **Assumptions** are often referred to as rules. They are your guidelines for how you conduct yourself. You also have rules for others. Examples of assumptions/rules: 'I should always complete a task' or 'Other people's needs are more important than mine'.

- **Core beliefs** are the deepest level of thought and are often quite rigid. Again you can have beliefs about yourself, such as 'I am likable' and beliefs about others, such as 'Others are trustworthy'.

Feelings
Feelings are also referred to as emotions or mood.

Behaviour
Behaviour, or actions, describe most, if not all activities - for example, working, resting, eating, driving and even sleeping. Avoiding certain activities also comes under this category, such as not going out to meet friends.

Physical reactions
'Physical' includes some of the following examples: your appetite being disturbed; sensitivity to the cold; pain; and changes in your energy level.

The diagram on the next page illustrates how these areas are interconnected.

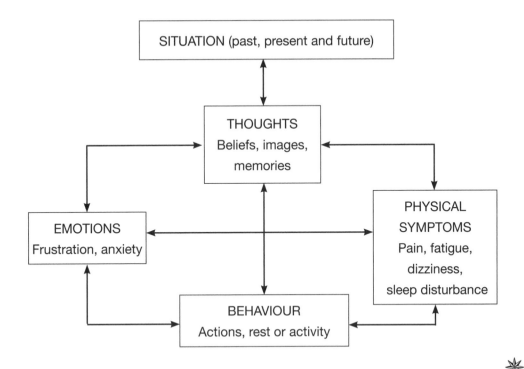

How do your thoughts connect with what is happening to you?

The term 'situation' can refer to anything that is happening in your life - for example, housing issues, work problems, relationships and practical concerns. It can also include events or situations in the past that have impacted on your thoughts and feelings. Most people with CFS/ME encounter practical problems - for example, managing working hours. There may be times when the reactions of other people can cause upset and difficulties. Look at the following situation.

Task

Life situation - You are unable to work full time due to your symptoms. A meeting has been arranged with your manager to discuss working part-time.

- Write down the different thoughts you might have in this situation.

- Write down how you feel in response to these thoughts.

Now compare your thoughts and feelings with the examples given below.

Possible thought	Emotional response
My manager has supported me in the past. He/she understands my situation. He/she will be open to the suggestion of part-time working	Calm
My manager will think I am not up to doing my job and will therefore sack me	Anxious

I will ask to work part time but really I am a failure for not being able to work my contracted hours. I might as well quit	Guilt
My manager thinks this condition is all in my head. He does not believe in CFS/ME	Anger

As you can see from this example, the way you think or interpret a particular situation will change how you feel. It is therefore important to be aware of your thoughts in response to different situations. We will look at ways to help you identify your thoughts later in the chapter.

How do your thoughts connect with your feelings?

In the examples above, each thought about the same event led to a different feeling or emotion. Whenever you experience an emotion, a thought has usually come first. Some emotions have been shown to be associated with certain thoughts. For example, people who experience anger often have thoughts about others treating them unfairly or causing them harm. People who are anxious tend to have thoughts related to threat or being out of control. Depression is frequently linked with thoughts about loss.

When you think about an event or situation the emotions you feel may change depending upon what you have focused on. This is often due to what are called **biases** in thinking. For example, you may only see the things that match your current point of view, not noticing other information that disagrees with this. Sometimes information is missed or disregarded. You do not do this on purpose. It is how your mind selects information when you are feeling a certain way. It is very easy to respond to the first thought that comes into your mind without checking the facts. The following examples may help you understand how a bias in your thinking can affect your emotions.

Example

You left a message on your friend's answer machine to give you a ring. A few days have gone by and your friend has not returned your call.

Possible thought	Thinking bias	Emotion
She is fed up with me ringing her; she doesn't want to know me any more	Discounting. You are focusing on the negatives and not thinking about the positive experiences you have had with your friend	Sad
She only wants to know me when she wants something	Distorted. Again you may not be looking at all the information; are there times this has not been the case?	Angry
She is probably busy and has not picked up her messages	None	Calm

In general, people do not stand back and consider the way they are thinking. We are not taught to question our thoughts and decide if they are biased or unhelpful to us. However, the CBT model recognises that we can all have unhelpful or biased thoughts at times and that these thoughts can cause us to experience unpleasant emotions. There are a number of ways to deal with this type of thinking. We will look at these later (see page 130 on how to challenge your thoughts).

Sometimes it may be hard to tell the difference between your emotions and your thoughts. For example, someone may say, 'I feel stupid'. On first sight this may sound reasonable; however, stupidity is not an emotion. Emotions or feelings are internal experiences, like feeling afraid, happy and frustrated. When you use expressions like, 'I feel stupid', it is the thought, 'I *am* stupid' that causes you to feel that way. The following table shows examples of confusing a thought with an emotion.

Example	Possible thought	Possible emotion
I feel a failure	I cannot do this, therefore I am a failure	Anxious, depressed
I feel useless	I used to be able to do all sorts of things for others; now I can hardly do anything for myself	Guilt

At times your emotions may be a reaction to the events that are happening in your life. These feelings may be completely appropriate. In these situations it helps to recognise your feelings, express them (which is covered in the chapter on 'Dealing with Others') and to look for ways to manage them. A number of suggestions to help you manage your feelings are given at the end of this chapter.

How do your thoughts connect with your physical reactions?

The chapter on 'Stress' highlighted the effect that thoughts can have on the way we feel physically. To illustrate this point further, imagine you are lying in bed at night and you hear a noise downstairs. Your first thought may be, 'I am being burgled'. Your heart starts to race, you feel butterflies in your stomach and your mouth goes dry. These physical changes are a result of you thinking you are in danger. Sometimes your thinking can create difficulties managing your CFS/ME and may, at times, increase your physical symptoms. This is mainly due to how you act in response to your thoughts. The next table has examples given by people with CFS/ ME and shows the link between their thoughts, actions and the physical effect on their symptoms.

Thought	Impact on symptoms
'I hate the illness'	Energy consuming - creates an anger response, increases adrenaline, saps energy
'I am never going to get better'	Heightens anxiety, hard to relax, saps energy
'I am going to carry on regardless'	Denies symptoms; therefore do not rest when fatigued; more fatigue
'I am not trying hard enough'	Creates even further pressure, adding to boom and bust
'Nothing I do helps'	Decreases motivation, lowers mood and decreases quality of life
'I am letting others down'	Increases anxiety, increases emotional arousal and lowers energy levels

Task

- Identify any of your thoughts about managing your CFS/ME.

- Write down any physical reactions you notice in response to either these thoughts or how you have to act because of your condition.

How do your thoughts connect with how you behave?

You now understand that how you think affects your emotions and physical feelings, so we will go on to look at the link between thoughts and behaviour/actions. Throughout the day we act in ways that have often become automatic and of which we are not always aware. Problems can start when you can no longer do things the same way that has always worked for you before. For example, imagine you have taken the same route to work for years, simply driving on auto-pilot. One day you cannot go that way. Now you have to think not only of a different way to get to work, but you may have to ask yourself if you have enough petrol, will the alternative route take longer, and do you need to tell others about the delay? This shows how one change can have a 'knock on' effect on your future actions and thoughts.

Managing CFS/ME requires you to deal with a number of changes in your life, such as altering your working hours or how you do household tasks. How you think about the changes you need to make will influence how you do this. The following examples show you the effect your thoughts can have on your actions and emotions.

Example 1 - Whilst you are doing an activity you get the following thought: 'I need to rest, but if I do I will never get started again'. This thought could stop you from resting and push you to more activity, leading to an increase in your symptoms. This could add to a sense of being helpless.

Example 2 - If you have previously been energetic, worked long hours and had little time for rest or relaxation, you get the following thought whilst you are doing a task: 'I should be able to do all this; I used to be able to. Unless I achieve all the things I have planned then I have failed'. These thoughts may make you keep going despite the fatigue, instead of resting. This would probably increase your symptoms and you may have to stop anyway.

Task

- Can you identify anything you do, or the way that you are dealing with a situation that is currently causing you a problem?

- Can you think of any particular thoughts you have about this? Write these down.

Summary of this section

Dealing with a chronic condition, like CFS/ME, will inevitably cause changes and losses in your life. These changes will naturally affect how you feel. The way you think about adjusting to these changes will determine what you do and how you do it. The CBT model has been used to show you how the four areas of thoughts, physical feelings, emotions and actions/behaviour link together. We have discussed how your thoughts about a situation can affect how you feel and behave, using different examples to show how one situation can lead to a variety of thoughts and emotions.

When is a thought unhelpful?

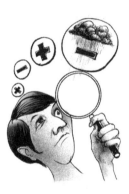

Identifying and changing your unhelpful thoughts forms a key part of using the CBT model. It is also important to adjust how you react to the various changes CFS/ME can bring. Next we will look at how to tell if a particular thought is unhelpful. If you are aware of unpleasant feelings or emotions, or find your reactions to a situation are a problem, it is useful to look at what you are thinking in more detail. To help you spot any unhelpful thoughts you can keep a thought diary. You will find an example of a thought diary on the next page.

How to use a thought diary

Column 1 - Write down what was happening just before the feeling started. Be as specific as possible. This may include: where you were, whether you were alone, what happened, what did you or others say? Did you have an image or particular set of thoughts before you felt the emotion?

Column 2 - Write down the emotion or feeling you experienced. It can be any emotion - for example, frustration, anxiety, contentment or anger. Alongside this, judge how intense the emotion was from 0 to 10 (10 being the strongest). This is to give you a rough guide.

Column 3 - To find any unhelpful thoughts, think of the words or pictures that went through your mind at the time. It may be useful to focus on any thoughts where you felt strong emotions, such as those that you scored between 6 and 10. Next are questions to help you know what you were thinking. This list does not cover everything and you may find some questions more useful to you than others.

Useful questions to ask yourself:
- Am I comparing what is happening to me now with the past?
- Am I thinking about the future based on how I feel right now?
- How do I view my body and what I am experiencing?
- How do I view what I am doing and how well I am doing it?
- How do I compare myself with others?
- What am I doing well or badly at the moment?
- How do I see myself?
- How do I see others?
- How might this (situation, physical feeling, emotion) affect my future?
- What do others think of me?

The more questions you can ask yourself the more likely you are to find the automatic thought making you feel or act this way. If it is difficult to find an image or memory that goes with your emotion, do the following. Imagine a time when you had the same feelings. Repeat in your mind images of this situation and allow your thoughts to drift. Be aware of any pictures you see appearing. Do not force an image; just let it emerge. Initially you may find it difficult to identify

MONITORING NEGATIVE THOUGHTS

Date	Situation	Emotion(s)	Automatic thoughts
	What were you doing or thinking about (refer to page 127)?	What do you feel? How intense is it? (0-10)	What exactly were your thoughts? How far do you believe each of them? (0-10)

your thoughts. It is not something that you are used to doing. As with any new skill, the more you practise finding your automatic thoughts the easier it is to pinpoint the ones that are causing your emotional response.

Some people find writing their thoughts down enables them to see how un-helpful or inaccurate they are. The process of writing the thought down allows you to put some distance between yourself and your thoughts. It can also help you to see your thoughts as thoughts. This may sound a bit odd, but sometimes you may react to a thought as if it is a fact. Just because you think something is true does not mean it actually is! An example is: 'I have achieved nothing this week'. It is common to focus on all the things that you believe you have not done; however, does this match the facts? You may have missed out some thing(s) that you did achieve. Sometimes information is discounted or missed, as it is judged not to be important. You need to check out all the facts before you make abso-lute judgements.

Summary of this section

We have now looked at how to find thoughts that may be unhelpful. Whenever you notice a change in the way you feel, check out what words or images went through your mind before you noticed the emotion. Remember we can all have unhelpful thoughts and react to them automatically. It is not easy noticing what is going through your mind. It takes practice. Next we will focus on challenging and changing thoughts.

How to challenge your thoughts

When you are confident in identifying your automatic thoughts and have prac-tised writing them down, you are ready to move on to the next stage. This is assessing them. There are several reasons why it is important to do this.

It helps you:

1.   to know what your words and expressions really mean.
2.   to notice any unhelpful patterns in your thinking.
3.   to work out how reasonable your thoughts are.

What do you mean?

Knowing the meaning of the words and expressions you use helps you to challenge them. For example, if you think of yourself as 'useless', what do you mean by this word? Would other people understand this word in the same way? Explaining the words and terms you use can show you if you are thinking in extremes. Describing them in detail helps you to see if these words or labels are unhelpful. Doing this gives you a better perspective on how you see yourself, others, or what is happening.

An example of this is, 'I'm a failure'. You may call yourself a failure when you have been unable to finish something. Think, what does this word mean to you? What is 'failure' and would you label someone else with the same word if they had done/not done the same as you? By doing this you can see how helpful or unhelpful your thought is.

This is called **All-or-Nothing Thinking**. It is a way of seeing yourself, others, or situations in the most extreme way, such as total failure or total success. When you are aware you are thinking in 'all or nothing' terms, define what the opposite would be. For example, what would you call 'success'? Would other people think the same? We will now look at more examples of common patterns in our thinking.

✳

How are you thinking?

We all judge the things that happen in our lives, past and present. It is common to react to these judgements as if they are based on fact. For example, at times you may feel that you know what another person is thinking or believe you know what is going to happen in the future? These thoughts are not a problem when they are positive - for example, when you think someone likes you or that you are going to have a great holiday. The problem starts when you see something in a negative way. For example, 'they think I am pathetic' or 'I will never be able to enjoy myself'. You cannot read other people's minds or predict the future. These types of thinking patterns are often called **thinking errors, thought distortions** or **cognitive biases**. When we are under stress, feeling ill or depressed, these thought patterns can become exaggerated and magnified, and thus start to affect our mood and actions. To help you to spot if you are using any thinking errors you can write down the ones you find in your thought diary.

For example:

Example	Description	Unhelpful thinking pattern
'They think I am pathetic'	You believe that you know what others are thinking, without having sufficient evidence for this	Reading other people's minds
'He's an idiot' 'I am useless' 'I'll never learn to relax' 'If I can't do all that I want to do, then there is no point doing any of it!' 'I have not completed the task; therefore I am such a failure'	You think in absolutes, as good or bad, black or white with no middle ground. You tend to judge people or events. You may condemn yourself as a person on the basis of a single event. This is common in people with CFS/ ME, who tend to have high standards	All-or-nothing thinking

'I walked too much yesterday. I have damaged my muscles by overdoing it. I will never get any better'	You tend to magnify and exaggerate the importance and meanings of events and how awful and unpleasant they will be, overestimating the chances of disaster; 'anything that can go wrong will go wrong'	Expecting a catastrophe
'It's my fault'	You take responsibility and blame for anything that happens, even if it has little or nothing to do with you	Taking things personally
'I will never be able to go on holiday; the distance is too far to travel'	You predict the future, and come to negative conclusions even when there are no definite facts. You may dismiss problem solving to deal with the situation	Jumping to conclusions
'My husband is angry with me because I am not well enough to go out. He does not care about my feelings'	You tend to focus on the negatives and ignore or misinterpret positive aspects of a situation. You focus on your weaknesses and forget your strengths; you always look on the dark side	Negative focus
'I must clean the house twice per week.' 'I should do things to a high standard.' 'I must put other people's needs before my own'	You tend to have fixed rules and unrealistic expectations, regularly using the words should, must and can't. This tends to lead to unnecessary guilt and disappointment. You may have adapted your rules due to the impact of CFS/ME - for example, 'I can't do it the same way because of the condition'. However, you may have put them to one side now only to go back to them whenever your energy returns	Living by rules

Looking for evidence

Knowing more about any patterns in your thinking helps you to stand back and question if there are any other ways you can view the situations you face. There are a number of techniques you can use to develop different thoughts – ones that fit the facts and are based on the right information. One method is to gather evidence **for** and **against** each thought.

For example: 'I have not done anything worthwhile today.'

Evidence *for* my thought	Evidence *against* my thought
I have been sitting in front of the television for most of the day	I did take care of the children, sorted out their breakfast and got their clothes ready for school
I have not washed my hair	I did make myself something for lunch
There is a pile of ironing still sitting in a heap	I have prepared the evening meal
I have not seen anyone today	

Once you have looked at the evidence both for and against your original thought, think about an alternative, more realistic, thought that takes everything into account. An example of developing an alternative thought based on all the facts is given below.

Automatic thought	Evidence *for*	Evidence *against*	Alternative thought
'I cannot pick up my children from school. I am a bad mother'	Don't pick up the children from school. School clothes not ironed. Don't invite their friends home. Don't go to the park	Spend time talking with the children about their day. Take an interest in what they do. Help them with their homework. Give them lots of hugs and praise	'I may not be able to do a lot of practical things with my kids, but I am caring, affectionate and show an interest in their lives. These things show I am a good mum'

Notice in this example you are not trying just to replace a negative thought with a positive one. You are coming up with a more rounded alternative rather than accepting the first thought that springs to your mind. Next are some more examples of thoughts that people with CFS/ME have found unhelpful and another way to think about them.

Questions to help you develop alternative thoughts

1. *Am I confusing a thought with a fact?* A thought is not a fact! Just because you believe something does not necessarily mean that it is true. Would other people accept your thoughts as correct? Would the thought stand up in court or be dismissed as circumstantial? What objective evidence do you have to back it up or contradict it?

  • **Automatic thought** – 'When I met Peter in the street, he didn't smile at me so I must have done something to offend him.'

- **Challenge** – 'It is true that he didn't smile at me but I have no reason to believe that he is upset with me. Perhaps he didn't see me or was thinking about something else – in fact, I've done that before myself.'

2. ***Am I jumping to a conclusion?*** This happens as the result of basing what you believe on your automatic thoughts rather than on fact. Remember that none of us is a mind-reader nor can we predict the future. Don't jump to conclusions – stick to what you do know and if it is troubling you, see what more you can find out.

- **Automatic thought** – 'I had some good days and bad days, but I don't seem to be improving, I will always be ill.'
- **Challenge** – 'I know the nature of the illness means that there are good and bad days. This does not mean that I will always be ill.'

3. ***Am I thinking in all-or-nothing terms?*** Everything is relative. People for instance are not usually *all* good or *all* bad. Are you being too extreme in how you view yourself, your skills, your assets or even your health?

- **Automatic thought** – 'I did that really badly – I might as well not bother.'
- **Challenge** – The fact is you didn't do it as well as you would have liked to. This does not mean that it was no good at all. If you always expect yourself to reach a hundred per cent you will very rarely be satisfied.

4. ***Am I using 'ultimatum' words in my thinking/thinking in absolutes?*** Watch out for words such as 'always'/'never', 'everyone'/'no one', and 'everything'/'nothing'. Usually the situation is not so clean cut. Think about words like 'some people', 'some things' and 'sometimes'.

- **Automatic thought** – '*Everything* is *always* going badly for me.'
- **Challenge** – 'This is an exaggeration. Some things go badly for me, as they do for everybody else, but some things can go well too.'

5. ***Am I concentrating on my weaknesses and forgetting my strengths?***
Often people overlook problems they handled successfully in the past and
forget about the resources they possess which enabled them to overcome dif-
ficulties. Ask yourself: 'How did I cope before?'
- **Automatic thought** – 'I would have done this in 15 minutes before; now
  I can't do anything well.'
- **Challenge** – 'Maybe it does take longer, but I still get the same outcome.
  I still have the skills, but I just have to adapt them in order to manage my
  CFS/ ME.'

6. ***Am I taking something personally that has little/nothing to do with
me?*** When things go wrong, we may assume that it is our fault, or that blame
may be directed at us, even if we had little or nothing to do with it.
- **Automatic thought** – 'Mary doesn't like me; if she did she would not
  have shouted at me like that.'
- **Challenge** – 'I know Mary was in a bad mood today and she told me she
  had had a fight with her boyfriend last night. Maybe she is just taking it
  out on me. She'll probably apologise – she did last time.'

7. ***Am I expecting myself to be perfect?*** Perfection is something that we
cannot expect ourselves to achieve. It is just not possible to get everything
perfect or to be correct one hundred per cent of the time. If we continue to
expect this standard we are bound to be disappointed. Accepting that you
are not perfect does not mean you have to give up on trying altogether. Learn
from your mistakes rather than being paralysed by them.
- **Automatic thought** – 'This is not good enough – I should be able to
  finish whatever I start.'
- **Challenge** – 'I can't always carry out everything I plan – I'm fallible just
  like all human beings. It would have been nice to finish it, but it's not a
  disaster that I didn't, and look at how much I did get done.'

8.   ***Am I using a double standard?*** You may be expecting more of yourself than you would of another person. How would you react to someone else in your situation? Would you be so hard on them? What would you say to them? Why aren't you being as kind to yourself as you would be to someone else?

- **Automatic thought** – 'I'm pathetic; I shouldn't get so upset by things.'
- **Challenge** – 'If someone else was upset by this situation, I'd be sympathetic to them and try to help them find a solution. There is no way I'd call them pathetic and in any case, doing so would not help the situation at all. I can apply these rules to myself too.'

There are more ways to challenge your automatic thoughts that we cannot cover in this book. If you are interested in learning more, there are some self-help resources listed at the end of the chapter. We will now look at things you can do to manage your thoughts and feelings and how to gain a better perspective on a situation or event.

Summary of this section

In this section we looked at different ways to challenge your thoughts. These included how to find thinking patterns that are unhelpful to you, looking for evidence for and against your thoughts and developing alternatives. This is not easy. It requires new skills and will only come naturally with repeated practice.

Testing things out

There will be times when you find it difficult to take on board another, more realistic thought. Even though the thought is based on fact and you know logically it makes sense, it somehow does not feel right. This experience is very common. There are examples throughout history which highlight these difficulties. Christopher Columbus found it difficult to recruit sailors on his ships to travel to the Americas, as the sailors still held the belief that they would fall off the earth. Even though he could demonstrate that the world was round through scientific evidence they found it hard to believe. Only when people returned from their voyages could they start to shift the way they had thought about the world. This same principle applies to everyday thoughts. We have a tendency to go back to our well worn patterns of thinking, particularly when we are under stress.

One way to help you to build confidence in your alternative thought is through action – trying out new ways of behaving; doing things differently. You may want to try out a new way of doing things to gather evidence to support or disprove your original thought.

For example

You may experience more fatigue in the evening and think that you could never make arrangements to go out with friends, because you would not be able to hold a conversation. You worry that people find you boring.

Here are a few options for how you could respond to this thought:

- React as though the thought is true and not go out, which may cut you off from your friends.
- Plan to go out with some friends still thinking this way and then write down exactly what you predict will happen. For example, 'People will not be able to understand what I am saying; they will look bored, sighing and looking away, not including me in the conversation.' Afterwards, go back to your prediction; did your thought fit the facts? Think about what you learned from *this* situation.
- Challenge your thought; come up with an alternative based on the facts. For example, 'I may be unwell so I will have to limit how long I go out for, but my friends will be pleased to see me. Just because I don't talk a great deal does not mean I am boring.' As with the previous option, write down your predictions of what will happen and then look at this afterwards.

When you are testing out new ways of dealing with situations remember not to view the new behaviour or way of doing something as either having worked or failed. It is about learning something new. You may want to repeat it a few times so you are confident in your new way of dealing with things. You may also want to adapt things along the way based upon what you have learned. Sometimes you may find out that your first thought was true and based on fact. It is helpful to see this as a problem to be solved or accepted, rather than becoming despondent about it.

For example
'Other people do not understand my condition and think I should get on with it'. Here are a few ways to deal with this thought.

- This thought may be true but why would that bother you? What does it mean to you? Answering these questions may help you to decide how to respond.
- You might want to think about the other person's attitude and to change what you do to cope with it. For example, know that others may be ignorant of the condition, but that you do not have to defend yourself. Accept that you cannot force them to understand and you can still do things to help yourself by managing your symptoms.
- You may want to tackle this reaction from others by being assertive (as explained in Chapter 8 on dealing with other people). Explain that they have their opinion but if they would like to understand the condition more you can get some information for them to read.

This is just one example of how to deal with information that matches your first thought. You may want to develop an action plan for a variety of difficult situations you regularly experience.

Most of the strategies within this chapter have focused on identifying and challenging your unhelpful thoughts. There will be times when you experience physical reactions or emotions that cannot be changed by doing this. For example, you may feel tense dealing with the demands of the day. At these times, acknowledge your physical or emotional state and share your feelings with others who are close to you. You can also cope with unpleasant physical feelings and emotions by focusing on another activity. Activities that require attention, such as crosswords and reading, can help as a distraction. This is because you cannot think or concentrate on more than one thing at a time. You may also find that relaxation is helpful. You have already read about the use of distraction and relaxation in relation to dealing with stress. Experiment with these various forms of activity until you find activities that help.

Summary of this section

We have looked at strategies to help you deal with situations that cause unpleasant thoughts, emotions and physical feelings. There may be many other approaches that you will find helpful with this. The main message is to experiment with different ways of doing things to assess which benefits you most. If something does not help the first time, try it again at another time before you completely dismiss it.

What to do next

You may have found that using the strategies we have described has helped you to deal with certain situations or problems more successfully. It is usual to find that after repeatedly challenging your unhelpful thoughts, other similar thoughts appear. This can happen when certain rules, assumptions or beliefs lie beneath the negative thoughts. To illustrate this, consider the following example. You have grown up in a family which had a strong work ethic; you remember comments being made that it is important to go to work even if you are ill, and sitting around when jobs needed doing was a sign of being lazy. You also recall being given praise for hard work. You may then have developed the following rules, although you would usually not be aware of this:

- It is important to be busy; if not it means you are lazy.
- Other people will not approve of you if you are not working.

If you hold such beliefs, then taking time off work or having time out to rest may bring up thoughts about what others think of you. You may be harsh or critical of yourself. Challenging the unhelpful thought gives you temporary relief, but to get rid of it you may need to tackle the rule or assumption behind it. This is beyond the scope of this chapter. There are a number of cognitive behavioural self-help books that can help you to address your assumptions and core beliefs, if you want to take this further. You may also wish to explore cognitive behavioural therapy from a trained therapist if you feel this approach would help you manage your CFS/ME and it is too difficult to tackle this on your own.

Managing your mood

What is depression?

Depression is a common disorder affecting one in five people at some point in their lives. Research has shown that rates of depression increase in those suffering from any chronic health condition. It is unsurprising, therefore, that rates of depression are also higher in people with CFS/ME.

Depression is a serious illness and is very different from just feeling sad or miserable. If you are depressed you are likely to have very *strong feelings of sadness* which last for several weeks or months. These feelings may interfere with your carrying out your day to day activities. This may be less obvious if you have CFS/ME as your level of activity will have reduced already. It may be your inability to do all the things you are used to which has caused you to become depressed.

Other symptoms of depression

- loss of interest in activities you used to enjoy
- stop experiencing any pleasure in your life
- lack of motivation to do anything any more

Other symptoms overlap with symptoms of CFS/ME, which is why if you have both conditions, they tend to make each other worse.

- fatigue and lack of energy
- sleep difficulties (especially waking up early)
- loss of appetite and weight
- indigestion, constipation
- changes in menstruation
- slowed movements and speech
- reduced interest in sex
- poor concentration
- hopeless and helpless about your situation
- more tearful than usual, crying at things which you would normally brush off
- feelings of guilt
- low self esteem
- feeling excessively anxious or worried
- more irritable than usual
- difficulty making day to day decisions.

For some people their symptoms are so distressing that they experience ideas that life is not worth living and may start to have thoughts of suicide. It is *extremely important* that you discuss these feelings, if you have them, with your doctor. If you suffer from CFS/ME and you are also depressed, it is even more important to seek help. Getting treatment for your depression will improve these symptoms and as a result make it easier for you to manage your CFS/ME.

Managing anxiety

What are anxiety disorders?

Everyone feels anxious sometimes. Anxiety is a normal and necessary feeling to have in our day to day lives. If we never felt anxious we would not recognise difficult or dangerous situations and might put ourselves at risk. Anxiety can be both psychological, (when you get lots of worrying thoughts about a situation), and physical (when your heart beats faster and you get sweaty and shaky).

Problems with anxiety can develop if you frequently experience anxiety symptoms for no apparent reason. Or if the symptoms you experience in difficult situations are so extreme that they stop you doing things that you want to do. This is when the normal experience of anxiety can become an anxiety disorder. Everyone with CFS/ME has to cope with stress and some people with CFS/ME develop anxiety symptoms alongside their CFS/ME symptoms. Others may have had problems with anxiety before developing CFS/ME but developing the condition may make their anxiety worse.

Generalised anxiety disorder

In this condition people often describe feeling anxious all the time. You may experience:

- feeling of tension in your body
- feeling that something bad is about to happen
- worrying thoughts about all sorts of situations and issues
- on edge and being unable to relax
- feeling more irritable, impatient
- become easily distracted
- problems with sleep due to the intensity of your worrying
- physical symptoms : dizziness, palpitations, muscle aches and pains, dry mouth, excessive sweating, stomach ache, diarrhoea, headaches.

This condition often starts quite gradually and there is not necessarily a specific event or time that you can pinpoint as the trigger. Not being able to identify the cause of the anxiety can make symptoms worse and some people begin to worry that there is no solution to this. This can become a vicious cycle, with anxiety levels rising further.

Panic disorder

Panic attacks are common; at least one in 10 people experience them occasionally. Panic disorder is a condition in which people have frequent panic attacks, usually for no apparent reason. This can leave the sufferer feeling very worried about when the next attack will be. People often describe a sudden onset of palpitations, chest pain, choking sensation and dizziness and feelings of unreality. At the same time there is often an intense fear of collapsing or dying, losing control or going mad. Individual attacks usually last for minutes, with a build up of symptoms which often result in a person leaving the situation they are in. If a panic attack occurs in a specific place (e.g. a supermarket or bus), the person may then avoid that situation in the future.

Although frightening, it is important to know that the symptoms of a panic attack will not actually lead to your having a heart attack, or cause you any physical harm. People who have had panic disorder for some time will often recognise the sensations they are having, and can learn how to control their symptoms.

Health anxiety

Health anxiety is a condition in which an individual becomes extremely preoccupied and concerned that the physical symptoms they are experiencing are caused by a serious health problem. They find it difficult to be reassured even after appropriate tests. Unlike panic disorder, there are often no sudden episodes of intense physical symptoms, although occasionally health anxiety and panic disorder do occur together.

If you become very anxious about your health, you may start to spend a lot of time checking your body for signs that something is wrong, maybe checking for lumps or skin blemishes. If you are not reassured by seeing your doctor about them, you may feel that doctors are dismissing you, which in turn may make you worry more. This condition can be very distressing and the effort of worrying, checking and seeking reassurance may impact significantly on your energy levels if you already have CFS/ME.

Treatment options

For both depression and anxiety disorders there are two main forms of treatment. These are physical treatments, such as prescribed medication, and psychological treatments, such as talking therapies. There are also a number of self-help options you can look at, particularly with anxiety disorders. These may be most appropriate if your symptoms are mild. If you think that you have a depressive disorder or one of the anxiety disorders, it is important that you discuss your symptoms and treatment options with your doctor early. These conditions need to be treated in their own right, rather than aggravate and worsen your CFS/ME symptoms.

Useful resources

- Dennis G, Padesky C (1995) *Mind over Mood - Change how you feel by changing the way you think.* New York: The Guilford Press
- Chalder T (1998) *Coping With Chronic Fatigue.* London: Sheldon Press
- Anthony MM, Swinson RP (1998) *When Perfect isn't Good Enough - Strategies for coping with perfectionism.* Oakland CA: Harbinger Publications
- Burgess M, Chalder T (2005) *Overcoming Chronic Fatigue - a self-help guide using Cognitive Behavioural Techniques.* London: Robinson

- Williams C (2003) *Overcoming Anxiety - A Five Areas Approach.* London: Hodder Arnold
- Williams C (2001) *Overcoming Depression - A Five Areas Approach.* London: Hodder Arnold
- Leahy RL (2005) *The Worry Cure - stop worrying and start living.* New York: The Guilford Press
- British Association of Behavioural and Cognitive Psychotherapists (www.babcp.co.uk).

David's story

When I first became ill with CFS/ME, I was unable to work for about two years. After practising grading and pacing strategies successfully, I returned to work part-time. I felt I was managing my condition alright by myself, until a retraining scheme was implemented at work which I found difficult to cope with. The feelings of anxiety I experienced built up over a period of time and I began losing confidence at work. I was making simple mistakes and struggling to adapt to the new ways of doing things. I was only working part-time when my colleagues were employed full time, so it did naturally take me longer to learn the new methods. I got into a downward spiral and I could not see a way out. My confidence was at the lowest I had experienced and I was anxious about lots of things. I was also feeling quite down about the situation. I noticed that my physical symptoms were closely linked to my emotional state and as I felt worse physically, my anxiety increased. That year I was off work through illness approximately 50 days.

The first step for me was to work on was why I was feeling anxious so much of the time. I was in work and I was doing as well as anybody else in my job. I began to notice that my thoughts were often about not being able to do a task and assuming therefore that I would never be able to do it. I worked on challenging my negative thoughts with more realistic ones, thinking that, although I might not be able to do the task immediately and it might take some time to learn how, it did not mean that I would never be able to do the work.

The process I worked on was being able first of all to identify what my thoughts were and then to challenge my negative thoughts. An example is, if I was given a piece of work to do, my immediate thought was to think I would never be able to do it or that I would do it and get it wrong. Once I could see what I was thinking, then the next step was to challenge those thoughts. In this example I could think that there is no reason why I would not be able to do that work, or that I would get it wrong when I did it. The secret for me was to believe the rational thought as opposed to believing the automatic one.

The benefits I experienced happened quickly for me. Even after a couple of weeks of working on noticing and then challenging my negative thoughts, I became aware that the number of negative of thoughts I was having was already less and I was believing, more and more, the rational arguments. Things turned around gradually and my confidence began to grow and my feelings of anxiety to lessen. My colleagues noticed and I was generally happier at work. I also felt better physically.

There was a knock-on effect into the rest of my life and, even though I was still only able to work part-time, I felt much happier and more relaxed about work and in control of the situation. I felt I had some control over my emotions, which in turn gave me some control over my physical symptoms.

I experienced some difficulties and I found that some thoughts were easier to challenge than others. My thoughts around work were easier to challenge than those in other areas of my life, simply because I had the opportunity every day at work to challenge them. I was experiencing feelings of anxiety in other areas of my life as well. I found it more difficult to turn other areas of my life around and the results took longer for me to see, because I was not able to work on these things every day as I was in my work life.

I know that working on identifying my negative thoughts and challenging them with rational arguments has benefited me because, after doing this work, I was absent from work only for 10 to 12 days a year, as opposed to the 50 previously. I think it is important to keep a sense of perspective and for me that means not panicking and projecting too far into the future. I work on concentrating on today, on the present, and I feel less stressed. I know it does not benefit me worrying about the future.

Another important thing is for me not to try to do too much all in one go. I need to focus on specific thoughts and feelings, rather than try to tackle everything all at once. I also know that attempting to block my thoughts does not work. I find that recognising my thoughts, acknowledging them and writing them down on a piece of paper, then challenging them and writing a realistic response to them, is a great way for me to support myself to believe the realistic response. A good analogy is to think about the ride at the fun fair that one person may feel is scary and another person may feel is exciting. The difference between the two people and their experience of the ride is the thoughts they are having about the ride. Also, this is not about positive thinking and denying negative thoughts. I know that attempting to block my thoughts does not work.

I have found it useful to write down what I have learned and to come up with a plan. I have written down the techniques I have worked on and how I can see I can use them in my life in different situations. I have looked at the thoughts and feelings that I have had in certain situations and have written about the success I have had when I have used the techniques. I have written down what might happen in a situation and what might not happen. To see the words written down has helped me not to panic. I also find it encourages me when I look back and see where I was and where I am now.

Chapter Seven

Memory and Concentration

Sue Stanley and Lisa Hinds

Introduction

People who have CFS/ME usually experience difficulties with mental fatigue and so have problems with memory and concentration. This chapter is designed to provide information about memory and concentration and how they can be affected by CFS/ME. It also aims to provide you with practical tips to help you to manage these difficulties.

Summary sheet

Topic	Read	Comments
Self-assessment		
Memory – what is it?		
A model of human memory		
Concentration – what is it?		
How memory and concentration are affected by CFS/ME		
Improving your memory and concentration		
Strategy checklist		

Self-assessment

Everyone varies in their ability to concentrate and remember, so it is important to start by reflecting on your own understanding and experience of memory and concentration.

Task

Think about the current difficulties or examples of problems that you are experiencing with your memory and concentration. It may help you to focus by writing these down.

Memory – what is it?

Sometimes people with CFS/ME are concerned that their brain is failing and that they may have a deteriorating condition, such as dementia. This can be very frightening. However, in CFS/ME the underlying problem is a lack of energy, leading to difficulties with concentration, which means information does not get stored in our memories in the first place. Therefore, when the symptoms of fatigue improve, the problems that people have had with their memories also start to improve.

To understand why you are having difficulty remembering even simple things, it may help if you start by understanding how your memory works. There are three main levels of memory and we are going to look at each of these in turn.

Sensory integration system

Your brain is constantly being bombarded with signals and information from both inside your body and also the world around you. However, your immediate memory has the ability to hold ongoing experiences in your mind only for a few seconds. Information from the senses (smell, touch, hearing, taste, and sight) are selected from your environment and filtered, perceived and organised by your brain. This system acts like a filter so that your brain does not have to deal with all the incoming information, all of the time.

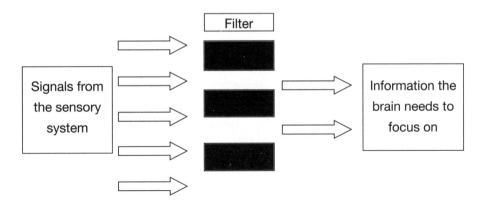

Your brain then needs to make sense of the new information. An example of this would be if you smell something the following may happen:

- Your olfactory system senses the smell, which is filtered from other smells in your environment.
- It is then 'perceived' – that is, your brain works out what it means - is it food or perfume? It also decides if it can recognise it, by comparing it to memories of smells from the past.
- If it is a smell that reminds you of something else, it will make more sense and be organised (filed) in the correct place.

Our immediate memory also provides us with an ongoing sense of being in the 'present'.

Short term or working memory

Short term memory decays quickly and has a limited capacity. For example, in order to understand this sentence you need to hold in your mind the beginning of the sentence as you read the rest. Loss of information from the short term memory can occur when there is interference. This is when new information displaces older information. Therefore, we often have the desire to complete the tasks held in short term memory as soon as possible.

The short term memory can hold only around *seven pieces* of information. Therefore researchers have noted that we remember things better in chunks, which is why a hyphenated phone number is easier to remember than a single long number. For example, the six figure number, 247569 could be written as 24-75-69. In this example, instead of having to remember six separate numbers (2 and 4 and 7 and 5 and 6 and 9) you are remembering just three numbers (24 and 75 and 69). Therefore, how information is organised or presented to your brain can determine whether it makes it through your memory processes.

Long term memory

As your brain is constantly being sent new information you have to pass the information to the long term memory or it will be lost. The long term memory is intended for the storage of information over a long time; days, weeks or even a lifetime. This is like a large filing cabinet in the brain for storing information. There are three parts to this:

1. **Storage**: Information from the short term memory is stored in the long term memory by rehearsal and repeated exposure. Therefore information is more likely to be stored effectively in your long term memory if you have focused on learning it or if you have come across it a number of times.

2. **Deletion**: Deletion is where you lose chunks of information from your memory or aspects of it become lost. It is mainly caused by decay over time and interference.

3. **Retrieval**: There are two types:
    • Recall: The information is accessed from the store of memories.
    • Recognition: The person knows the information presented but they have difficulty accessing it from the store.

All of these stages have to be completed for us to have a memory of an event. The more times you take information through this process, the stronger the memory becomes. For example, if you often think back to a particular happy memory from childhood, and try to recall as much detail about it as you can, the stronger that memory becomes.

The diagram below illustrates how all the stages link together for your memory to work.

A model of human memory

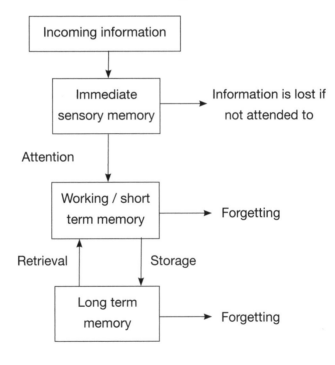

Concentration - what is it?

Concentration is the ability to focus our thinking in the direction in which we want it to go. We all have the ability to concentrate some of the time, but this can be affected by many things. In CFS/ME the ability to filter out necessary information from other thoughts or environmental distractions presents most of the difficulty. So you may find that how well you are able to concentrate changes, and that factors such as being in a noisy room or someone talking next to you, can destroy your ability to focus.

Task

It is important to start by being aware of the different factors that can affect your ability to think or concentrate. Identify physical, mental, emotional, environmental and situational factors that can impact on your concentration. If you are able to, write down what makes it easier or harder for you to concentrate.

Easier to concentrate	Harder to concentrate

Your ability to concentrate depends on a number of internal and external factors:

- **Your physical state**: In addition to the impact that fatigue has upon your mental processes, many of your other physical symptoms, such as pain, nausea and dizziness will also interfere with your ability to focus on one thing.

- **Your emotional state**: When you are in a rested, relaxed and comfortable state, your emotions tend to be calm, and you will be more likely to be positive about things. This makes you more able to concentrate. Conversely, other emotions, such as fear or distress, can have a negative impact.

- **Commitment**: We need to make a personal commitment to put in the effort needed to do a task. If you start in a half-hearted manner or feel reluctant about doing a task it is much more difficult to sustain your concentration.

- **Enthusiasm**: If you are interested in and enjoy doing a task it is usually much easier to motivate yourself to concentrate on it.

- **Skill**: Knowing how to do something gives you confidence, so you do not worry about your ability to do it. New tasks will therefore always require more effort to concentrate on them and you may, initially find them more difficult.

- **Environment**: There are lots of external factors, which can affect your ability to concentrate e.g. noise, temperature, being comfortable or being around other people who can 'stress you out'.

How are memory and concentration affected by CFS/ME?

Energy is needed for brain activity and as fatigue increases, this will affect your thought processes. Often people with CFS/ME describe experiencing a 'brain fog' following a period of time working on a mental task.

Your ability to remember depends on whether the information has been stored in the first place. So, have you been able to concentrate on the information presented to you in order for it to get into your short term memory and then be successfully filed it in your long term memory? If the senses are overwhelmed with information, the brain will find it more difficult to organise memories and they may not get stored in the right place or not even get stored at all.

Remember: even sitting in a room doing nothing uses energy as the systems of the body are still working. People often describe how their minds are still active when they are doing nothing - this will still use up vital energy. A common problem is that people focus on the physical energy that they are using and forget about all the internal demands for energy, including thought and mental processes.

Improving your memory and concentration

Strategies you may find helpful

Firstly, do not compare how you are now to your previous levels of ability. Human beings are typically only able to concentrate effectively for approximately 20 minutes at a time. However, many people look back at the past and focus on how good their cognitive skills were, often ignoring the times they got things wrong! Do not expect yourself to be at the same level that you were at in the past; be realistic.

The following strategies for managing difficulties with mental activities can be helpful.

Grading

* Apply the principles of grading to concentration and memory. For example, you might set yourself smaller goals, such as starting with reading half a page and, when this is manageable, increase it to three quarters of a page.

- Plan ahead; make sure you are not excessively mentally fatigued before focusing on an activity.
- Prioritise your tasks.
- Take regular breaks. It will help if you stop an activity before you become too fatigued; set time limits on doing mental tasks.
- Change activities regularly; it will help if you 'mix and match' tasks; swap from a mental to a physical activity.
- Focus on one thing at a time.

Environment
- Make sure your environment is suitable. Consider:
  - Lighting: is this at a suitable level?
  - Temperature: do you feel too hot or too cold?
- Think about whether there are people distracting you in your immediate environment, or if you are able to overhear people further away. Can you change location?

Resources
- Keep lists as they may help you to remember and prioritise tasks.
- Use diaries and calendars - put them in a place where you will see them regularly and get into the habit of checking them.
- Use sticky notes and fridge magnets to leave reminders in a visible place.
- Use a dictaphone to record ideas that you want to come back to later and then listen back to this at a more convenient time.
- Use your answer phone. It can be useful to screen calls that you may not want to respond to immediately. Leave these until you are ready.
- Put a message book by the phone - use it as soon as you have finished a call. Feedback messages when on the phone, in order to clarify and check you have the correct information. Do not be afraid to ask someone to pause for a moment while you write things down.

- Rehearse and repeat things you want to remember – either verbally or by writing them down.

Expectations of yourself and others

- Do not set your standards too high.
- Share responsibilities, for example, for remembering dates and events.
- Delegate: if someone wants to help – let them.

Starting to apply these strategies in your life

Many people are concerned about improving their physical fitness level but forget that it is also possible to work on improving mental abilities as well. However, this is an important area to focus on, as many people report being more distressed by their mental difficulties than their physical limitations. Our ability to think and make decisions is such a personal experience. People with CFS/ME often say that they no longer feel like themselves because of the loss of these skills. Therefore, it is important to include strategies for improving memory and concentration within your own rehabilitation programme.

In the next section we are going to look at how you apply the ideas that have been discussed to your daily life, in order to make it easier to concentrate and reduce the energy you spend on mental tasks.

Task

Complete the table overleaf, listing any mental activities that you want to achieve. Then, look back at the strategies in the previous section to identify which might help you with each particular task.

Task I want to concentrate on...	I can improve this by...

Strategy checklist

> ## Task
> DON'T GIVE YOURSELF A HARD TIME! Apply a practical strategy - see if it works for you. Below is a list of the techniques contained in this chapter. The columns on the right allow you to tick off the techniques you have tried and record if you have found them helpful. For most people it is a combination of factors that can help to improve their memory and concentration.

Grading

	used	helps

Setting small achievable goals

Take regular breaks, to prevent increasing fatigue

Change tasks regularly, using 'mix and match'

Focus on one thing at a time

Resources

	used	helps

Keeping lists

Using diary or calendar

Answer phone/ message book

Rehearse – repeat things you want to remember

Write things down you are trying to remember

Environment

	used	helps

Lighting

Temperature

Getting away from distractions

Expectations of yourself and others

	used	helps

Not setting standards too high

Sharing responsibility

Delegating

Useful resources

- Gross R (2005) *Psychology: The science of mind and behaviour* 5th Edition. London: Hodder and Stoughton

Ruth's story

I was diagnosed with CFS/ME in 2002. One of the symptoms I have experienced is difficulty with my memory and concentration. In particular, I have problems with word recollection. I find that this problem is worse at times of the day when my energy is at its lowest. I often feel frustrated by it.

When I was first diagnosed I reduced the amount of physical activity I was doing. To compensate, I increased the number of cognitive tasks I undertook. I began learning about managing my symptoms. One of the things I learned is that I need to be disciplined with myself. I learned that it benefits me to limit the amount of time I spend on cognitive tasks. To begin with I limited the time to 15 minutes and then I took a break. I knew I could manage to do 15 minutes without worsening my fatigue. The tasks I did included reading, writing, working on my computer, researching into CFS/ME and managing my finances.

I discovered that I benefited from varying my activities. Initially I would spend 15 minutes doing a cognitive task, then take a break. I would then go on to do a physical activity. Over a period of two years I worked at increasing the length of time I spent doing a cognitive task. I also worked on increasing the number of cognitive tasks I did in one day. By the end of 2006 I was able to return to work. I began by working for two hours per week, gradually increasing the number of hours. For me, as with physical activity, grading is important.

One challenge I have encountered is to do with the expectations I put on myself. I can easily over-do it and I have to work at monitoring myself. I use an egg timer which I set at the start of a task to tell me when to stop. I don't always stop when the timer tells me to! However, more recently I have noticed that I now get up about two minutes before the alarm goes off to turn it off! At work

I have some software on my computer that I can set to switch my computer off when I choose.

I have had to relearn the ways in which I work and the expectations and beliefs I have about myself. For example, I used to think it was rude not to concentrate one hundred per cent in meetings. Now I accept that in some tasks I will not be able to apply myself as much as I could. I allow myself to be tired and I accept that some tasks are not important.

I have created my own alternatives for certain words that I find difficult to remember. For example, my dog's lead is her belt and her collar is her necklace! I don't know why I find those words easier to remember, but I do. It does invite a few surprised looks from people at times.

I am aware that my energy is low in the late afternoon. This means I schedule meetings and challenging discussions for other times. I find working from home supports me to manage my time, energy and symptoms. I choose to keep my health problems to myself and so working from home means people are not as aware of them. Although I do not want people to know about my illness, I feel upset when people don't accommodate it.

I find writing lists supports my memory. I have to be careful not to set myself up to fail by writing lists that are unrealistic for me to achieve. When I first began working to improve my memory and concentration, I was recommended to read a newspaper. I decided to read the *Financial Times*! Now my husband and I fight over the tabloid papers. My husband says I have two speeds - stop and very fast. It is great that he supports me to slow down sometimes.

Chapter Eight

Dealing with Others

Ian Portlock

Introduction

CFS/ME is often referred to as 'an invisible illness' because you cannot see the symptoms. This may make it difficult for you to communicate with others about your condition and how it affects you. It can also make it difficult for others to understand your illness. This chapter focuses on the role of communication and how you can influence others' perceptions and responses to you, through how you communicate.

Summary sheet

Topic	Read	Comments
Can other people understand CFS/ME?		
Asking for help		

How you communicate with others		
How to be more assertive		
Know your rights		
Assertiveness techniques		
Dealing with criticism		

Can other people understand CFS/ME?

One of the commonest problems that people with CFS/ME describe is that other people find it hard to understand the condition. They struggle with how they can get other people to appreciate the effects that CFS/ME has on their everyday lives. People with CFS/ME often raise the following points:

- CFS/ME has traditionally been given unhelpful names such as 'Yuppie Flu', which have influenced people's perception of this illness, including those who suffer from it. People are faced with the stigma of this.
- CFS/ME is often misunderstood and wrong assumptions are made about the condition.
- Advice given by others is often not based on knowledge and understanding of CFS/ME.
- Other people's attitudes can often seem unsympathetic.
- People with CFS/ME often feel they have to justify and explain their illness.
- People with CFS/ME sometimes feel apologetic and guilty about their illness.

In cases where people are just ignorant and unknowledgeable about your condition, providing them with some education or written information about CFS/ME can help their understanding. There is information in Chapter 11 on 'Carers' that describes the impact of the condition. It is important to remember that the choice rests with you as to who you might give the information to and how much you want to share about your problems.

However, understanding is not all about knowing facts. There are many people who can be caring and supportive of others, without having any knowledge of the facts relating to the medical condition concerned. When you know people who are ill, do you need to have the full details of their symptoms and medical treatment before you can empathise with them? Someone's ability to relate to other people is often about their attitude and ability to listen. Sadly, some people will not change their views no matter how many research articles and reference books you show them about CFS/ME!

Just remember that no one can fully appreciate what it is like to have a problem until they have had it themselves. Did you understand what it was like to have CFS/ME before it happened to you? However, there are ways in which you can help people to understand it. You may put on your best 'face' when you are around other people and not show them how you are really feeling. Unless they are telepathic, how are they supposed to know? This is why how you communicate is so important in helping others to understand.

✳

Asking for help

You may find it difficult to ask for help. However, energy conservation is an important part of the management of your condition. It may be that those closest to you want to help but do not know how. You may have been very independent and self-sufficient in the past. Therefore, you are not used to asking others for help.

To enable you to start asking for help and to minimise unreasonable demands from others, you can use the following strategies. You may find it difficult at first, but they have the opportunity to be helpful in the long run:

- Communicate your abilities and limitations.
- Explain about the fluctuating nature of your CFS/ME.
- Accept help.
- Delegate.
- Postpone some tasks.
- Prioritise tasks.
- Learn to say 'no'.
- Learn to ignore ignorant or offensive remarks from others.
- Ask for support from those close to you.
- Include close family/friends/partners in your management plan.

How you communicate with others

The next section of this chapter describes different styles of communication. It is important to recognise that everyone uses these different communication styles. Many people are unaware of using them and the effects they can have. If you recognise what you are doing, then you can make constructive changes.

It can be difficult to change the way you communicate with others. However, if you change how you are communicating, this will influence how other people respond to you. It can be worth it. It can improve your relationships and help you manage your illness more effectively. If you need further support with becoming more assertive or need to discuss any feelings this raises, you can contact a local health professional.

Communication styles

Communication styles are the different ways in which people relate to each other. This section of the chapter looks at four different communication styles: direct aggression, indirect aggression, passivity and assertiveness. Most people use all of these styles at some time or another. On occasions they can be beneficial - for example, if you are angry you may get what you want, and sometimes letting others have their way can help relationships run more smoothly. However, if you frequently use direct aggression, indirect aggression or passivity, as your way of communicating, it can have a negative effect on your relationships and on you.

CFS/ME and communication styles

Communication styles can be important in relation to your condition, not only in terms of affecting how you manage it, but also because they can have a direct impact upon your energy level. If you frequently use an aggressive style of communication it can be very draining on your energy. This is because your body's response to communicating in an aggressive style is similar to your stress response, which was covered in Chapter 5 (pages 95-98). Your heart beats faster, your muscles are tense and energy is rapidly used up. This leads to an increase in your fatigue.

If you frequently use a passive style of communication it can also increase your fatigue. If you are passive you may find it difficult to limit your activity levels when others ask you to do something. This may lead you to push yourself beyond your baseline. This in turn leads to an increase in your fatigue.

Very few people use one style of communication all of the time. For example, some people can be assertive at work and passive at home, or vice versa. You may have found that you are more likely to use an aggressive style of communication since developing CFS/ME. This may be due to the fatigue and frustration you experience as a result of the condition, and the attitudes of others towards you. Alternatively, you may find it difficult to be assertive with others. For example, you may realise that you have used an indirectly aggressive approach to help you get rest when you feel you need it.

This chapter goes on to discuss assertiveness. This is a style of communication which helps you express what you want, balanced with the needs of others, and so helps you to reduce your fatigue. The next few pages describe each communication style in turn, so you can understand more about them.

Passive communication

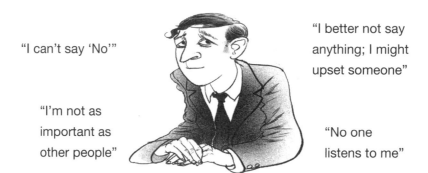

"I can't say 'No'"

"I better not say anything; I might upset someone"

"I'm not as important as other people"

"No one listens to me"

This style of communication comes across to others as submissive, helpless, indecisive and apologetic.

Advantages and disadvantages of passive communication

People with CFS/ME commonly say that they feel more passive after developing the condition. If you are passive you may feel unable to say no, and therefore do tasks for others which will decrease your already low energy levels. Other advantages and disadvantages to this style are contained in the table on the next page.

Advantages	Disadvantages
Often others are kept happy, because they get what they want.	You do not get your needs met.
You avoid conflict, which means you avoid the uncomfortable feelings it might provoke and conserve the energy it might use.	You may not feel others appreciate you and you can start to resent them.
You can see yourself as a nice person.	You can increase stress and therefore fatigue levels by trying to keep others happy.
You can avoid taking responsibility for your own life and leave decisions to others.	You have no way of changing the behaviour of others if you are unhappy with it.

Aggressive communication

"Do it my way or else"

"I don't take any stick from anybody!"

"Oh for X@!*"X sake!"

"Just get lost and leave me alone"

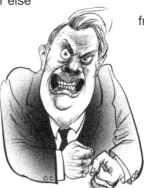

"If I want anything done properly I have to do it myself"

"You're hopeless"

This style of communication comes across to others as bossy, bulldozing, opinionated and overbearing.

Advantages and disadvantages of aggressive communication

If you are directly aggressive this can increase your stress and can lead you to experience increased fatigue.

Advantages	Disadvantages
You can get what you want	You may get a defensive or aggressive response from others and not get what you want
You can release anger and get issues 'off your chest'	Others may begin to dislike and avoid you
You can blame others	You do not take responsibility for your own issues and blame others instead. Therefore the issue may not get resolved
You can defend yourself against other people who are being aggressive towards you	You may feel guilty after being aggressive

Indirect aggressive communication

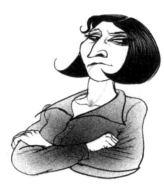

"Don't be so sensitive. I was only having a laugh?"

"I don't get angry. I get even"

"Don't you worry about me. I'll just sit here and suffer"

"She would have done it for me. Why can't you?"

This style of communication comes across to others as sarcastic, manipulative, ambiguous and guilt-inducing. This is less easily detected than direct aggression. If someone uses indirect aggression towards you, you may feel you are the one at fault and experience guilt, unless you know that the other person is using this communication style.

Advantages and disadvantages of indirect aggressive communication

If you are indirectly aggressive your feelings remain suppressed. Consequently, you may continue to feel tense, which will increase your fatigue. Also, the issues you are concerned about do not get resolved, which further increases your fatigue.

Advantages	Disadvantages
You can get others to do what you want them to do	Others may begin to resent you if they realise you are manipulating them
You can pass the blame onto others and you do not have to take responsibility for the problems in your life	It is stressful and fatiguing to 'keep up' this type of behaviour. Having always to think 'one step ahead'
You can avoid being overtly aggressive	You will not get the best out of relationships with others if they are based on manipulation instead of communication

Assertive communication

"I have equal rights with other people"

"I'm responsible for my life"

"I'm not perfect, but nobody is"

"No, I don't want to do that"

"I feel upset about the situation"

This style of communication comes across to others as direct, positive, accepting, honest, spontaneous and responsible.

Advantages and disadvantages of assertive communication

If you are assertive this enables you to say 'No' and limit the amount you do for others, in a way that is acceptable. This helps you to manage your condition. You may have to use energy in the short term to address the problem. However, you will reduce the anguish and worry that the situation may cause over the longer term and so you will use less energy overall.

Advantages	Disadvantages
You can communicate what you want and balance your needs with those of others.	You may feel uncomfortable changing your communication patterns.
You are responsible for yourself and you are able to change the things in your life that you are not happy with.	You may experience increased stress to begin with if you have not been assertive before.
You can plan and organise your life, helping you and those around you to manage your condition.	
You will reduce your stress, which in turn will increase your energy level.	You may find it difficult to change your communication style if you have frequently used aggressive, passive or indirect aggressive styles in the past.

How to be more assertive

Being assertive is an effective way to relate to others. Communicating assertively will help you to avoid misunderstandings and resolve issues more quickly.
Assertiveness is a way of communicating your *feelings, rights, needs and opinions,*
whilst taking into account those of others. This can be a balancing act. It is
important to remember that being more assertive will reduce stress, tension and
internal conflict. All of which are a drain on your energy.

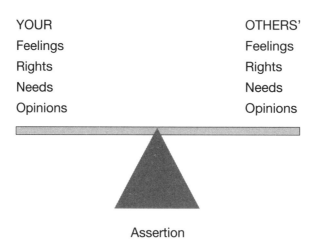

YOUR   OTHERS'
Feelings   Feelings
Rights   Rights
Needs   Needs
Opinions   Opinions

Assertion

Being passive

If you put other people's feelings, rights, needs and opinions above your own,
you may come across as passive. You can be taken advantage of by others,
whether they mean to do so or not. You may also find yourself having to work
hard trying to keep others happy. They may not appreciate what you are doing
and the impact this has upon your CFS/ME. This can lead you to push yourself past your baseline and spend all of your energy doing things for everyone
else.

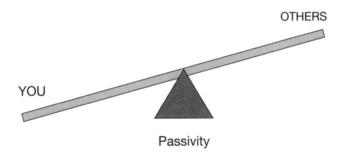

Passivity

Being aggressive

If you disregard others' feelings, rights, needs and opinions, you may come across as self-centred and aggressive. This is draining on your energy levels and seldom leads to you getting the result you want. Sometimes people can feel angry about having CFS/ME and the losses they experience in their life. This may then come across in how they communicate, making other people withdraw from them.

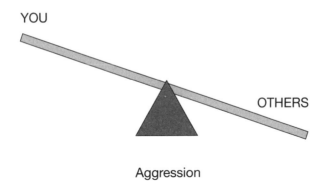

Aggression

Know your rights

To be assertive you need to recognise that you have certain reasonable rights within your relationships. If you do not believe that you have rights then you will not be able to stand up for them. You have the *right* to be treated with respect as an equal human being and to make your own decisions. You have the *right* to express your opinions, thoughts and feelings and to be assertive. You have the *right* to be listened to and be taken seriously. You have the *right* to say that your needs are equal to those of other people and to choose not to be responsible for others. You have the *right* to change your mind and to make mistakes.

> **Useful questions to ask yourself:**
> • Do any of these rights stand out for you?
> • Do you feel that you could assert your rights more often?
> • Would there be any problems if you did this? How could you resolve these?

Assertiveness techniques

This chapter contains a number of techniques that can help you to be more assertive, rather than passive, aggressive or indirectly aggressive, as a way of helping you to manage your CFS/ME.

Saying 'No'

Many people have problems saying 'No' to others. This can sometimes lead to them taking on too much. As you have CFS/ME, taking on more commitments may exceed your energy supply. A consequence may be an increase in your fatigue and other symptoms. If you feel guilty about saying 'No', bear in mind that if you manage your energy now and do not go past your limits, you will support your recovery. It will then be more likely that you will be able to help others in the future. The following outlines ways of saying 'No' assertively and confidently, without feeling guilty.

Saying 'No' Assertively

- Be straightforward, but not rude and you can make your point effectively.
- Tell the other person you are finding it difficult.
- Tell the other person what your needs are.
- Ask for more time.
- Do not apologise and give elaborate reasons for saying 'No'; it is your right.
- Remember it is better in the long run to be truthful than to cause frustration and resentment within yourself.
- You are entitled to change your mind about things that you have already agreed to.

Scripting

Scripting is a technique to help you plan what to say to someone in a difficult situation. The advantage of scripting is that you can work out what you want to say beforehand, and because you have CFS/ME writing this down can help you to remember what you want to say at the time. It works best in situations where you know that there is an outstanding issue that you want to discuss with someone. As you become familiar with the technique, you can also use it during conversations, as problems occur. The following describes the technique, which is based on the phrase 'Even Fish Need Confidence'.

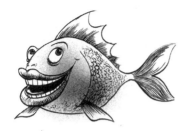

EVEN	**F**ISH	**N**EED	**C**ONFIDENCE
V	E	E	O
E	E	E	N
N	L	D	S
T	I	S	E
	N		Q
	G		U
	S		E
			N
			C
			E
			S

1. **EVENT** – Be clear about the situation or behaviour you would like to talk about, as it may have been some time since this happened. The person you are talking to may be thinking of something else when you start the discussion.

So your script may start with " About…" then state the event or situation

2. **FEELINGS** – No one can argue with your feelings, but they can with your opinions. When you use 'I feel' statements and are honest about your feelings, people are more likely to take notice. Beware if you can say "I feel *that*…"; it is probably a thought not a feeling!

So use the words " I feel …" and check that you have stated your emotion. For example, "*I feel* upset when you tell me it's all in my head". If the other person keeps taking you off the point, just keep repeating your feelings until they start to take notice. Then carry on with the next two stages.

3. **NEEDS** – Once you have their attention tell them what specific action you are looking for.

So start with " I need…" and tell them what you need or you want them to do.

4. **CONSEQUENCES** – How will life be different if they change their behaviour? How would it make you feel and how might it be of benefit to them?

So state if this happens, "then…" and describe what difference this would make.

Task

If you would like to practise this technique in a situation that is relevant to you, please complete the sheet below. You can use this format to help you prepare to discuss an issue with another person and it will help you to be more assertive.

Event

Feelings

Needs

Consequences

Repetition / Broken record

Using this technique will prevent you from being sidetracked from what you would like to say. This is about using calm repetition, over and over again. This enables you to maintain your position without falling prey to manipulative comment, irrelevant logic or argumentative bait. In the times before CDs, a broken or scratched record would play the same line of a song over and over again. If you apply this principle to a message you would like a person to take note of, you repeat the important point of your argument or your 'core message' over and over again.

Example

Peter: 'Jane, can you take me to the supermarket in the car because it is raining?'

Jane: *'I am unable to take you right now, Peter'*

Peter: 'But it's raining and I need to do a big shop. You know I would do the same for you'

Jane: *'I am unable to take you right now, Peter'*

Peter: 'It will only take 20 minutes'

Once you have made your point, if the other person is not listening, you can acknowledge their point of view, but keep repeating your position – for example:

Jane: 'I know it wouldn't take that long, *but I am unable to take you right now.* You can borrow my umbrella if you like?'

Peter: 'Okay then, I'll catch the bus'

Notice how Jane kept to her broken record technique. Note also how Peter attempted to throw in a 'red herring' – *'I would do the same for you. It will only take 20 minutes'.* This is an irrelevant issue and is an attempt to distract Jane from her point. The more you practise, the easier it becomes. Do not worry too much about what the other person's potential response might be. You are making a reasonable point.

Other assertiveness skills

Here are descriptions of some other strategies that you can use.

• Be specific
Decide what it is you want or feel and communicate this specifically and directly. This skill helps you to be clear about exactly what you want to say. Avoid unnecessary padding and keep your statement simple and brief.

> **Example:**   Peter: 'Can you cook tea tonight, please.'
> Jane: *'I'm too fatigued to manage it today.'*

• Fielding the response
In order to communicate effectively, indicate that you have heard what the other person is saying. Do not get 'hooked' by what they are saying. This skill allows you to acknowledge their response and continue confidently with what you want to say or ask, without feeling defensive or aggressive.

> **Example:**   Peter: 'But I've had a busy day at work.'
> Jane: *'I know you've had a busy day at work, but I really am too fatigued to cook tea tonight.'*

• Workable compromise
Compromise is important when there is a conflict between your needs and those of someone else. Assertiveness is not about winning. Negotiate from an equal position. This means finding a true compromise which takes the needs of both of you into consideration. Compromising on a solution does not mean compromising your self-respect.

> **Example:**   Jane: *'If you cook tea, I'll do the washing up,'* or *'We could order a take away if you prefer?'*

•Self disclosure
Sometimes it is helpful to disclose your feelings with a simple statement - for example, 'I feel nervous' or 'I feel guilty'. The immediate benefit is to reduce the anxiety you may be feeling, enabling you to relax and feel more in control.

Example: Jane: *'I feel guilty about not being able to cook tea'*

• Process not content
This technique is about focusing on what is happening in the situation, rather than the content of what is being said. It helps you to take a step back and comment on what is happening in an objective manner and prevent both of you being stuck in your own points of view.

Example: Jane: *'I think we are tired, hungry and frustrated. I'll order a take away and we can talk about this when we have calmed down'*

Dealing with criticism

One area that everyone can find difficult is coping with criticism. When people have CFS/ME, this can affect self-esteem and confidence, so you may feel more sensitive to any criticism. Negative comments about you from other people can leave you feeling hurt and upset, whether this was their intention or not. The following strategies help you to deal with criticism, depending on the type of impact that it has upon you. Some comments may not really bother you, whilst others may touch on things that you value highly about yourself or are sensitive about.

Negative assertion
This skill allows you to handle hostile or constructive criticism from others that you see as irrelevant. By agreeing with and accepting criticism, if it is appropriate, you need not feel totally demolished. Instead of reacting to criticism as an accusation, you can feel less defensive and become more accepting of yourself. However, be careful to distinguish between what you *do* agree with and what you *do not* agree with (see 'fogging').

Example: Jo: 'You wouldn't be too tired to cook tea if you had not spent all afternoon working in the garden.'

          Alex: 'You're right. I probably did over do it in the garden today. I'm sorry I didn't plan ahead very well.'

Fogging

This is useful when you agree with part of a statement, but do not accept it in full. The idea is to talk as long as possible around the subject, and include within this the part that you feel is right and also the aspect you do not agree with. The longer you can keep talking, the more likely someone else is to get bored and move the conversation on.

Example: Jo: 'You wouldn't be too tired to cook tea if you had not spent all afternoon working in the garden'

          Alex: 'You're right. I probably did over do it a bit in the garden today. I probably didn't plan ahead very well, but it was a lovely day and I don't get to go outside very often, so it seemed like a good idea at the time, but you never know how these things are going to work out, ...'

Negative enquiry

This is the best response to use when the criticism that you are being given is unfair or upsets you. It enables you to challenge the criticism by making the other person defend what they have said and give you evidence for it, rather than just leaving you feeling bad. It also encourages the other person to express their own negative feelings directly and leads to a general improvement in honest communication and understanding. You simply ask *why* they have made that comment.

Example: Jo: 'You're useless'

          Alex: '*Why* do you say that?'

Summary

Remember the golden rules of dealing with other people

- **Assertiveness = yours and others'** needs, rights, feelings, opinions
- **Remember your rights**
- **Practise your techniques** - scripting, broken record, saying 'No', etc
- **Assertiveness** can lead to a saving in physical and mental energy.

Lisa's story

At the start of the illness I was unaware how dealing with other people used my energy and that even an emotional reaction about a person or situation did this. I have always been a high achiever and I was concerned by what other people thought about me. When I was first ill I made a lot of assumptions about what I imagined other people were thinking. I did experience some people's misunderstanding of what CFS/ME is and some of those people were among those close to me. Some people were not sympathetic and told me that I looked 'ok' and that everyone gets tired. When those people visited I pushed myself to carry on as I had before I was ill. I cooked for them, took care of them and those people were getting the impression that I was ok. They did not see me in the weeks before their visit, when I rested and prepared. They did not see me in the time after, when I had to stay in bed for a couple of weeks to recover. I often found myself not addressing issues that came up with other people at the time they arose. I would be upset and go over things in my mind, sometimes for weeks and months afterwards.

Other people's reactions were very significant to me and it was having a big impact on my life and my symptoms. I was wrapped up in feeling guilty, seeing the illness as my fault and I was continually pushing myself to keep going. I felt guilt for not being able to do as much as I previously had at home and that meant my husband had to do more. I was so ashamed about not working and being at home, that I would sit with the blinds closed so that people couldn't see me. I imagined they would be wondering why I was at home and not working. I assumed they would think I was lazy and didn't want to work. I have now accepted that the illness isn't my fault.

One technique I now use is to prepare for any situation that I feel might be difficult. I think in advance about what I might say to the person involved. I have also learned to explain to other people what the illness is all about. Although my parents were sympathetic, even they could not fully understand why sometimes I wasn't able to go to a family gathering, for example. I worked on explaining the illness to other people. I found that if someone cared about me they would listen to what I had to say and adapt to me and being around me. One of the most challenging things I have had to accept is that some people do not want to listen and will not accept what I am saying. There are still those who see the illness as a weakness or a reason for not doing things. I am learning to be assertive and let people know what I can and can't do. I still feel hurt when someone doesn't understand. I now know that all I can do is explain and I can't do anything to *make* other people understand, if they are not willing. In the past I could have spent months being upset about someone's negative reaction and now I know I can let it go. I still sometimes feel angry towards people who do not understand and I feel it is healthier to feel anger towards them, than blame myself and feel guilty.

In the past, I would often say yes to someone who asked me to do something even though I did not feel well enough. Now, I feel more able to talk to that person about how I will feel tomorrow, if I do what they want me to do today. I explain to them that if I rest today, it is likely I will be well enough to do something tomorrow. I still, sometimes, feel that they might be thinking I am making an excuse for not wanting to do something.

I have always tried to keep doing some part-time work throughout my illness. One of the most challenging experiences I have had is to say no to work, when they asked me to do some extra work when I was not well enough to do it.

I have found that by saying 'No' and being more assertive I am not using as much energy as I was when I was getting upset. Also, I am not dwelling on upsets as I did in the past. By being more assertive, I am in control of my life and how I manage my time each day, so that I am managing my energy much better. I go to work two days a week and so I have to ensure that I do less, on the day before I go to work and on the day after I have worked. Being assertive means I do not over-commit myself on those days.

I still find it difficult sometimes to tell other people that I have CFS/ME and I know that they will either understand or they won't. If they don't there is nothing I can do about it. I now realise that I am not responsible for making everyone else happy and I don't have to live up to what I think are their expectations of me, which may or may not be true.

Chapter Nine

Physical Activity and Exercise

Penny Forsyth

Introduction

Exercise is a factor that influences the amount of energy within the human body. People with CFS/ME often struggle with the idea of exercise, or they may have had a negative experience with prescribed exercise. Research over the last few years has shown that exercising at the right level has significant benefits for CFS/ME sufferers, but what is the *right level* for you?

Summary sheet

Topic	Read	Comments
Exercise and CFS/ME		
Will exercise make me worse?		
What happens if I do very little physical activity over a long period of time?		
Getting the balance right		
The importance of posture		
How do I start?		
Making decisions about exercise		

Exercise and CFS/ME

Exercise can be treated like any other physical and mental activity and can be undertaken in a slow and graduated way. Research evidence in the last few years supports the use of graded exercise in the treatment of people with CFS/ME, but the way that you do this is very important. It is known that exercise increases overall body fitness. This applies to people with CFS/ME, as well as those who do not have the condition. Other benefits include lifting mood, reducing anxiety and aiding mental clarity, probably by reducing stress. However, because of the nature of the condition, you need to think carefully about how this can work for you.

What do we mean by exercise?

Exercise refers to a part of physical activity that is structured and focused on improving your physical fitness. Physical activity is any bodily movement in which you use your muscles and which needs an increase in energy to do so.

The benefits of physical activity/exercise

The benefits of physical activity and exercise on the body are well known. Exercise helps to:

- Maintain muscle strength.
- Prevent heart disease.
- Prevent circulation problems.
- Maintain lung function.
- Maintain bone density.

Exercise can produce positive responses in the body due to releasing *endorphins*. These are neuro-transmitters, which act as pain killers, lower blood pressure and can give you a feeling of happiness.

What sort of exercise is appropriate in CFS/ME?

Exercise is an emotive word and can conjure up a variety of images in people's minds, from a gentle stroll to vigorously 'pumping iron' at the gym. Some researchers have looked at the benefits that people with CFS/ME can experience when using graded exercise, as part of a treatment programme. However, you exercise your muscles everyday, in ways that you do not always think about. Daily activity of any description, from getting dressed and preparing meals, to DIY and gardening, can be considered exercise, as you have to produce extra energy and use your muscles to do them. Exercise does not have to be something that you do in addition to all the other activities you have to manage within your energy levels.

Useful questions to ask yourself:
- What activities do I do now which exercise my muscles?
- Are there are any of these that I could do differently or use as part of a graded approach to help my health?

If you feel you are ready to return to additional sport or exercise on top of your daily activity, then gentle exercise initially, such as a walking programme, using a graded approach, can be helpful. It has been suggested that the best level of graded aerobic exercise tolerated by people with CFS/ME is between 40-60% of maximum heart rate. That is at a moderate level, where you start generating body heat but you are able easily to carry out a conversation, speaking in full sentences. This level is normally achieved at a steady even walking pace, which makes regular walking one of the most accessible means of taking exercise.

Will exercise make me worse?

If you think of exercise as any physical activity that causes you to increase energy demand above your normal daily level, then you can apply the same principles of *pacing* and *grading* that you do to other activities; this has been described in chapter one. You can use graded exercise as part of your daily routine, so that it fits in with the other demands that you are dealing with. People often report that they become worse if they push themselves to increase their exercise level each day, without considering all of the other things that still need their energy. Exercise can be a means to gradually improving physical fitness, increasing wellbeing and reducing fatigue levels in the longer term, but take a balanced approach.

It is important to start at the level that you can manage consistently. For example, if you can manage walking for two minutes every day, then that would be your starting point. However, if you can only manage two minutes on your 'better' days then this would not be a good place to start. You can use the task on page 33, to help you to work out your baseline.

If any form of exercise, even at the lowest possible level, causes a *significant increase in symptoms* then seek professional advice, or concentrate on managing other aspects of your fatigue, until you are at a level where you can start to introduce more exercise safely.

What happens if I do very little physical activity over a long period of time?

The effects of prolonged inactivity on the body have been well demonstrated. It has been found that after just 24 hours of bed rest, your body's ability to maintain normal blood pressure in response to activity reduces. Also, your heart rate increases and sympathetic nerve activity to muscles reduces. Muscles become significantly weaker within a few days of continuous bed rest. The consequences of prolonged inactivity are that a person will have added difficulty returning to normal levels of activity. This will add to the existing problems caused by CFS/ME.

An example to illustrate this would be a runner who is used to running 10 miles a day suffers from a hamstring injury and is forced to rest during recovery. She does not return to 10 miles a day straight away. If she did attempt the 10 miles she would suffer breathlessness and a racing heart, and the next day would have sore and painful muscles.

A similar thing happens to a person with CFS/ME following a period of bed rest or inactivity, even after just walking around the house. It can also take longer with CFS/ME to recover back to the level you were at before the deconditioning than it would take for an unfit runner to return to his previous performance level. This is because, in addition to overall deconditioning, you must take into account all the other factors which influence your fatigue levels. This can be done by using an activity diary, described in chapter one.

How might this make you feel when you start to increase your physical activity?

- You may feel your muscles are weak and notice a loss of muscle bulk.
- You may feel dizziness after lying flat for too long, due to poor control of your blood pressure.
- You may feel weak, unsteady and have aching in your muscles after initial attempts to exercise.
- You may notice more fatigue, lethargy, chronic pain and mood changes.
- You may feel loss of balance.
- You may find your weight has increased, adding strain to your joints and causing pain.

Getting the balance right

The best approach for anyone, including the runner and the person with CFS/ME, is to build up physical activity gradually, within limits that they can sustain over at least five days per week. This level has been found to be most effective for increasing overall fitness. In addition, it is important to balance this physical activity with other demands on your energy levels and not to exercise at levels that cause you to spend more time in bed, for the reasons we have described. Often people choose a level that is too high initially and feel downhearted when they cannot achieve this consistently.

A certain level of muscle ache after an increase in exercise level is considered a normal response, as muscles are stressed from being worked. This, however, should subside after three to four days as muscles become stronger.

On the other hand too much exercise/activity can be followed by a relapse, so a balance between rest and activity is needed.

The trick with this balancing act is to know your own limitations at any given time, so judging the difference between the amount of activity or exercise that is beneficial for you and overdoing it. Unfortunately, no one can tell you if an

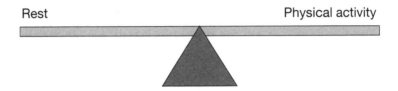

Rest   Physical activity

exercise or activity is going to be too much for your present levels of energy. The only thing to do is to try something. Normally people with CFS/ME set their standards too high, so always start on the low side of what you think you should do. If it causes excessive symptoms, rest until recovered and then have another go, doing a little less. Learn to recognise your warning signs and your current limitations. Bear in mind that your energy level and your ability to carry out activities will fluctuate, as this is the nature of CFS/ME. Once you have found a manageable baseline level of activity, you can very gradually increase this.

Example: Use a gentle walking programme, beginning with a minute or two each day. If this is manageable, with no additional effects, slowly increase the time. Increase by small amounts initially - for example, by thirty seconds. (This is only an example. Select an activity that is meaningful to you and begin at a level that fits with how you are at the moment.)

The importance of posture

Normal or 'good' posture is important in maintaining your flexibility and your ability to move normally. This helps you to maintain your activity levels. Good posture acts to protect the body against abnormal wear and tear and also helps prevent acute muscle injuries. Good posture also makes the most of the mechanical efficiency of your body when you are doing daily activities and enables you to move using less energy.

Does posture matter if I have CFS/ME?

The answer to this is YES, IT DOES! Your body is built for moving and to bear weight in gravity. This is why your muscles, bones and joints are only able to maintain themselves in response to active movement. People in industrial societies tend to lead more sedentary lives. Those who have CFS/ME have added difficulty in maintaining physical activity levels and so their bodies may be more vulnerable to postural problems. The positions you adopt when you have fatigue, or difficulty moving, may not be helpful in the longer term. If you have to alter the way you move in order to deal with physical problems – for instance, avoiding putting weight on one leg due to pain – it may be helpful to see a physiotherapist.

What is normal posture?

The spine is comprised of three curves, which enable mechanical efficiency. The size and shape of these curves is influenced by genes, body build, weight, use and condition of the joints and muscles. The three main curves are at the neck, at the back of the chest, and in the lower back. *Normal* posture comprises these three curves, with shoulders held loosely enough to enable them to swing slightly while the pelvis 'hitches' each hip in turn, as a person walks, so transferring weight from side to side. The head is held up but not pushed forward, as this will increase the curve around the neck and create strain.

What can I do about poor posture?

Your lumbar curve makes the biggest difference to your overall posture, because you mainly sit, lie down or do activities in a standing position. Also, because your muscles become easily fatigued when they are held in one position, known as *static posture*, such as standing or sitting without support, you may tend to slump within a minute or so. 'Slumping' when sitting, which is when your lower back flattens out and you become a 'C' shape, puts extra pressure on your vertebral discs and strains the pain-sensitive structures that lie behind them. This position, if prolonged or repeated, often contributes to back pain. The good news is that you can prevent this by using some firm support when you are sitting - for example, if you use a folded towel to help maintain the curve in your lower back. A folded towel is preferable to a cushion, which tends to squash down. Avoid standing if you can; if you do have to stand, some movement is better than prolonged standing in one fixed position.

How do I start?

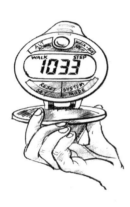

While a steady baseline will help you to feel more in control of your energy levels, life rarely allows us to balance energy in and out precisely! Ask yourself how much exercise you do currently. You may need to keep a diary or think about the physical activity you do regularly. If your fatigue levels are high and you are currently doing little physical activity, think about using a pedometer to measure how many steps you take each day. Monitor these numbers for a fortnight. This will give you an idea of how much you walk day to day.

If this varies, you may need to take the lowest number of steps as your starting point, and then gradually increase it. The idea is to reduce the 'boom and bust' type cycle in physical activity. Slow, gradual increases in your physical activity, when you are ready, are more likely to improve your physical fitness. Regular exercise can, also, increase feelings of wellbeing. People with CFS/ME often find that, provided they use a gentle graded approach, these benefits are also felt in other areas of their life. If you are in doubt about how to approach this, we suggest that you discuss this with a specialist.

Starting to stretch

Stretching your muscles can be a useful place to start doing a little more exercise, or in conjunction with a planned walking programme. Stretches need to be carried out when the body is warm - that is, not first thing in the morning but once the body has 'got going' with some movement. Stretches are not appropriate if you are very immobile at the moment. You can get advice on safe stretching from a professional.

Making decisions about exercise

Many activities involve some aspect of physical movement. One of the best ways to gradually increase physical demand, before you start to take any additional exercise, is to increase the activities that you do already, everyday. This can be done by increasing:

- Frequency
- Duration
- Resistance (making the task a little harder)

Before starting to exercise, plan what you will do. It is important to consider your current exercise tolerance.

Useful questions to ask yourself:
- How much do you do now?
- How often?
- How different is your current level from what you plan to do?
- What is the best time of day for you? Some people feel better in the morning; others are better as the day goes on.

Before beginning, think about clothing, footwear, hydration levels, personal safety, and what you would like to do! Remember to warm up, and cool down. Stretches are useful when the body is warm. Think about the other demands you have on your energy, both physically and mentally, as these will influence your available energy. Remember, using a diary may be helpful.

Summary

We hope this chapter will encourage you to think about how you might incorporate a small amount of gentle regular exercise into your daily routine. Remember, it does not matter how low the level is. It needs to be at a level you can do almost daily without impacting too much on your new balanced lifestyle. If you have any difficulties, stop and ask to be referred to a specialist for individual advice.

Useful resources

- Burgess M, Chalder T (2005) *Overcoming Chronic Fatigue: a self-help guide using cognitive behavioural techniques.* London: Robinson
- Campling F, Sharpe M (2000) *Chronic Fatigue Syndrome (CFS/ME) - the facts.* Oxford: Oxford University Press
- NICE (National Institute for Clinical Effectiveness) (2007) *Chronic Fatigue Syndrome / Myalgic Encephalomyelitis (or Encephalopathy): diagnosis and management of CFS/ME in adults and children.* London: NICE

Lee's Story

I have been involved with sport all my life and, in the two years prior to becoming ill with CFS/ME, I completed a number of endurance challenges, including the coast to coast walk and the Pennine Way. I was training three times a week, completing sessions of 20 minutes on an exercise bike, followed by 20 minutes' running on the treadmill and 20 minutes on the rowing machine. I also enjoyed walking and it was on a walking holiday in the Lake District that I first noticed something was wrong. I was part way into a planned 12 mile walk and I had to turn back because I was experiencing symptoms of dizziness, aching muscles and a lack of energy.

At the start of my illness, because I did not understand what was wrong, my natural tendency was to try and push through it. I remember pushing myself to complete a 50 minute gym session and then spending the next three days in bed exhausted. In the early stages there were some days when I wouldn't go out of the house, because I couldn't walk very far. I could only manage to read one page of a novel before I was exhausted and had to stop. As time progressed, three or four months into the illness, I was able to walk to the local shops, which were about 10 minutes' walk away. I would walk there, have a rest and a drink and then walk back. The severity of my symptoms varied. There were some days when I couldn't go out of the house and there were other days when I managed to do a little gardening. I could do about 10 minutes of light gardening, such as watering or dead-heading. I was resting every day and, sometimes, I would simply lie on the sofa and on other days I would have the radio on and listen to the cricket. I was pleased when the test match was on because it was something to listen to and kept me occupied. I needed a lot of rest, so I spent approximately three quarters of the day resting. At that time I was sleeping for about seven hours a night and it was intermittent, broken sleep. In the morning I did not feel rested and would wake up feeling tired.

I started employing the technique of grading my activity. I began at a very low level and increased it by small steps, after consolidating each step before taking the next. My starting point was to walk for 10 to 15 minutes at a time and there were some days when I could manage only five minutes. It did vary and I had to listen to my body. There were some times when I could do a little more and there were other times when I had to rein myself in and not do as much. I stayed at this baseline level for about a month before attempting to increase it. I increased the time I spent walking by increments of between two and five minutes, small amounts, approximately every two weeks. I then moved on to exercising on the rowing machine, which worked better for me than walking because I was not carrying the weight of my own body. I increased the amount of time more slowly on the rower, by approximately two minutes each time. Then I consolidated that for several weeks before increasing it further. I wasn't working initially and then I worked part-time hours.

The challenge for me was my own personality. I am someone who will keep going and, through the sport I have taken part in previously, I have learned to keep going and not give in. I discovered with CFS/ME that this approach only makes things worse. I had reached a level where I could manage 20 minutes on the rowing machine, then on one particular day I was feeling great and decided to continue rowing after 20 minutes. I actually spent 40 minutes working on the rowing machine that day. I knew I should have stopped at 20 minutes and I didn't; my old way of doing things took over.

One of the benefits of doing some physical exercise whilst suffering with CFS/ME was having a sense of control over an illness which I often felt was controlling me. From time to time, I got it wrong. I worked at learning from those mistakes because I paid for my over exuberance. I learned to be disciplined with myself.

Currently I am much recovered and back to working full-time. I am experiencing a busy time at work, which often involves me working long hours. I am being sensible and have cut back on the amount of exercise, because work is making greater demands on my energy than normal. I am still doing some physical activities and spending time in the garden. I can now manage heavier work, such as digging, regularly exercising on the rowing machine, one or two times a week for 30 minutes at a time. I feel I could do more, but currently with my other commitments, that is enough. In the summer I went on another walking holiday in the Lake District and walked for three out of the four days I was there.

It has taken me 18 months to get to where I am now from being able to walk for only five minutes a day. It has not been a smooth progression; sometimes I have taken a step forward and then a step back. By managing my activity and exercise, I have gained a sense of being in control of my life again and that I can still do the things I love doing, although maybe not as vigorously as I did them in the past. The key for me has been getting the balance right. There is no simple answer and I know that I have to listen to my body. Over the course of my illness there have been some days when I have felt ok and that I could do some exercise. There have been other days when I knew I could not exercise. There have been a lot of days when I had to make a judgement call and decide if I was well enough to do some exercise. Often on those days I decided to attempt some exercise and reduce the amount or intensity of it. In the short term, I sometimes felt that activity and exercise took away from my energy reserves but what I realised was that, by building up activity and exercise levels gradually, they added to my energy reserves in the long run. I also worked with not simply increasing the time I was doing an activity or exercising, but the intensity, frequency and type of activity and exercise I was doing.

Chapter Ten

Relapse and Setbacks

Sue Pemberton

Introduction

CFS/ME is a difficult condition to manage and predict, as it can have a fluctuating pattern and can change over time. That is why people with CFS/ME can find it so frustrating. You may have a good day and believe you are getting better, then go on to find you have more bad days. Learning how to manage the times when your condition seems to be getting worse, or not improving, is an important part of the recovery process. This chapter will help you to identify what may be triggering a relapse and the strategies for dealing with these difficult times.

Summary sheet

Topic	Read	Comments
Recovery		
What is a relapse?		
What can cause a relapse?		
Relapse plan		
Common reactions to relapses		
Hints on coping with relapses and		
Setbacks		
Stuck on a plateau		

Recovery

When will I be better?

This is a hard question for anyone to answer. There is a spectrum of severity with the condition. Some people can have mild CFS/ME and can still do some activity, whilst other people are severely affected and unable to go outside. So equally, there is also a spectrum of recovery. Some people feel they recover to the point that their symptoms no longer stop them doing things, whilst others feel that their symptoms are not changing. Most people find there is an improvement in their symptoms and an increase in their energy levels. However, this can be a slow process and requires making small changes over time.

What is 'better'?

You may think of yourself as *'well'* when you can do all the things that you used to do. However, in learning how to manage CFS/ME, you may have realised that the way you used energy and lived your life in the past is no longer the best way for you to maintain your health and energy levels in the long term.

A healthy person will still have fluctuating levels of energy, with days when they do not feel as well or energetic as others. The human body needs times when it can relax and recharge, as well as having times when it is active. Many people who develop CFS/ME led very active lives before their illness and were used to being 'on the go' all of the time. Therefore, as they recover from the condition, their natural tendency is to fall back into pushing themselves to do too much. They may forget about the habits of pacing and looking after themselves, which they previously used to help them to improve.

It is important to look after your energy at all stages of recovery. Think about what you want to do as you get better. Are you wanting to go back to how you were before, or aiming for a new, more balanced lifestyle?

> **Useful questions to ask yourself:**
> • Imagine that you have been able to wave that magic wand and all your symptoms have gone – what would your life be like?
> • Think about how you would be using your energy. Do you think this would be a healthy lifestyle for the long term?

What is a relapse?

The fluctuating nature of CFS/ME will mean that you experience times when your symptoms seem to get worse. This is part of the 'boom and bust' pattern of the condition. However, there will also be times when these dips seem to be more severe and last for longer than you expect. People often refer to this as a *relapse* in their symptoms. As recovery happens, people often report that the relapses they experience are not as severe and recovery becomes quicker.

What can cause a relapse?

Sometimes a relapse occurs and you can find no reason why this has happened, but often you can identify possible triggers for it. This can be helpful, as it can enable you to prevent a future relapse, or reduce the severity of it, by trying to minimise the trigger factors. It can be useful to make a list of the sorts of demands that you were dealing with before the relapse happened. This will help you to see if there have been any changes, or a build up of events, that may have tipped the balance. In this way you can learn how to anticipate when you might be susceptible to having a relapse, such as when you are facing a life change or increased stress or demand. Then you will be able to take action to prevent this happening again.

Main causes of relapses or setbacks

There can be many different triggers for a relapse but some common examples include (adapted from Macintyre, 1998):
- Physical exertion beyond your limits, for either that day or sustained over a few days.
- High levels of mental demand and/or stress, for example, having to focus intently on a task, taking a test, or meeting deadlines.

- If you experience a viral or bacterial infection, e.g. cold / flu, tooth infection, urine infection, etc.
- Other changes in your health, such as hormone changes, developing other medical problems and increased allergic reactions.
- Emotional stress / demanding life events - for example, divorce, bereavement, family illness, changing jobs, moving house, or getting married.
- If your mood becomes low.
- Physical stress or trauma - for example, after surgery, accidents, or injury.
- If you have changed or stopped taking a medication you usually take, or as a reaction to a specific medical intervention.
- Lifestyle factors, such as drinking alcohol or changing your diet.
- Environmental factors, such as high noise levels and travelling.
- Extreme changes in climate, such as winter cold and the lack of daylight.
- If you stop using the management techniques described in this book and revert to your previous patterns of coping.

Symptoms that are caused by doing too much activity can develop within a few hours or over a few days. If you find it difficult to identify what triggered a relapse, then keeping a diary may be helpful. If you have a relapse please use the following exercise to help you to work through it.

Relapse plan

Task

Make a list of things that have changed in your life or the differences in your normal routine or daily activities that may be related to your relapse.

Are there any on-going things that are stopping you recovering from this relapse?

What things helped to improve your fatigue previously that you could use again now? (For example, using activity diaries, reviewing your diet, improving the quality of your rest, being assertive with others)

What do you think you need to do next?

Common reactions to relapses

People may handle a significant deterioration in their health in different ways. Some of the common responses that people talk about are:

- **Taking preventative action**
  'I knew that I had a cold so I made sure I looked after myself, rested up for longer than I would have done in the past and then gently started to do things again.'

- **Back to square one**
  'I panicked to start with because I just thought that I was back to square one again. I felt so frustrated and fed up that I went to bed, feeling so ill and couldn't face trying to do things again. Then I realised that this wasn't going to help me, and that I knew more about how to manage my CFS/ME than I did when I first got it. I couldn't be back at the beginning again.'

- **Living in a box**
  'When I had a bad relapse I thought I must have overdone it and that must be the limit of what I should be doing. Afterwards, I avoided doing certain things and just lived within my limits. The problem was life was very dull. I felt like I was living in a box and I didn't think to test my limits again. It was much later that I realised maybe I could do those things again; I just needed to be more careful and maybe go about it differently.'

- **Finding the culprit**
  'To start with, whenever I had a relapse I thought it must be due to having a virus, because that is what happened when I first got CFS/ME. Then I realised that different things seemed to affect me, and sometimes it was a combination of things. I started to think about what I could do about this, rather than thinking it was a virus and just waiting for it to go away.'

- **Going back to the books**

    'When I think I might be having a relapse I get all the information I have back out again and re-read it. I then remember all the things that I had forgotten to do because I had been feeling better. It just helps me to think about what I need to do to get back on track again.'

Hints on coping with relapses and setbacks

There are many things that you can think about when you have a relapse. The following may be helpful:

- Managing setbacks is part of recovery. Do not blame yourself, but see this as an opportunity to actively manage the situation. You may notice that your symptoms are improving when the relapses you experience become less severe and you recover more quickly. Ask yourself, if given the possible triggers, this relapse could have been worse? Recognise what you have done to deal with this.
- Do something about your problems as soon as you recognise them. It will take you less time to get back on course again.
- Start at the beginning. Re-read the information in this book on grading your activity and taking planned rests, for example. Think about what has helped you before and use this again.
- Prioritise your activities. Remember, do one thing at a time. Give yourself the time you need to convalesce.
- Are you expecting too much of yourself at this present moment? Give yourself a chance; praise yourself for what you have achieved.
- Balance your days, as much as possible, with tasks, leisure and relaxation.
- Keep diary sheets again and establish what your current patterns are regarding activity and energy levels. Next, look at establishing goals and a realistic programme.

Stuck on a plateau

Another common problem can be that things are not going backwards, but they are not going forwards either. This is often described as being *'stuck on a plateau'*. Sometimes it is actually helpful to stay at the same level for a while. This helps the body to consolidate what it can manage before handling further increases in your activity. However, it can also become frustrating if this continues for a long time and progress seems to have stopped.

Common reasons for plateaus

- **Taking too big a step**
  There is too big a step between what you can currently manage and the next level up. So, whenever you try to increase activity it always fails. Think about making your increases smaller for a while; an example may be only adding on a minute at a time. This may just help you to get over that step and then progress may move forward quicker again.

- **Lack of stimulating activity and pleasure in your daily routine**
  Sometimes people have cut so much out of their lives in order to manage the symptoms that what is left is dull and boring. You need to have interest and enjoyment in your life, to give you the motivation and energy to be active. Is there one thing you could put into your week that you could manage and really want to do, even if it does mean having to rest more or reduce other activities around this?

- **Lack of direction**
  Sometimes people improve to a level where they start to think that they could do a little more, but they do not know what to do. They may have had goals in the past related to work or family that they know are unrealistic now but, because they have not thought about new, more realistic goals, they get stuck. Think about the things that interest you and that you enjoy. How could you work towards activities related to these? Many people have found voluntary work or courses at local col-

leges useful as a step towards this. You can usually start with only a few hours and there can be more flexibility, if you are not able to stick to the commitment each week.

- **Happy with our habits**
  Some people have got used to the limits of their condition and got into habits of how to do things in a way that doesn't increase their symptoms. To move recovery forward can be hard work and requires concentrated effort on balancing and increasing activities. For some people it is easier to go with how they feel, or what they have got used to, and making further changes seems a daunting task. However, these changes do not happen just by waiting for them. It might be helpful to think back to a time before you became ill, when you wanted to do something new in your life, or do more of something, for example, increasing your fitness. You would have needed to decide how you wanted to do it, plan what needed to change (such as making time for it) and be prepared to push your body slightly to do more in achievable steps. When you did this you probably found it worthwhile. In CFS/ME the principle is the same, but you may need to make the steps smaller.

The important thing to remember is that you have strategies, which got you to where you are now and they can also help you to climb further. Sometimes it is when people look back that they realise they have made more progress than they thought. Others have made this difficult journey and so can you.

Useful resources

- Burgess M, Chalder T (2005) *Overcoming Chronic Fatigue: a self help guide using cognitive behavioural techniques.* London: Robinson
- MacIntyre A (1998) *M.E.: Chronic Fatigue Syndrome - a practical guide.* London: Thorsons

David's story

I became ill with CFS/ME in 1994. The course of my illness was a series of ups and downs, with periods when I felt reasonably well and periods when I relapsed. I noticed that the relapses became progressively worse and after each relapse I found I could do less than after the previous one. After 12 years of ill health, I had reached a point where I was desperate to look at why I was experiencing relapses. Also, I wanted to know what I could do to avoid them and how to manage them when they occurred. I wanted to understand what was motivating me to keep doing things the way I had always done them and how I could learn to do things differently.

I know that there have been specific events in the past which have triggered relapses. One of those times was when I was due to move from Somerset to Manchester, to begin a new job. I found looking for somewhere to live and organising a move to a new city, two hundred miles away, very stressful. I became more and more anxious about the move as it grew closer. I wasn't sleeping properly and I was feeling churned up and sick. Those symptoms got worse the closer I came to the moving date. I know now that the relapse had begun before I moved. When I arrived in Manchester I put my things into my new home and drove across the Pennines to my parents' home in Leeds. I stayed with them and I never actually started that job. I realised that something which triggered a relapse in me was anxiety. So being able to recognise and manage that anxiety was something I knew I could work on.

A second relapse was triggered when my brother-in-law became ill and had to go into hospital, at the same time as I started a creative writing course at college. My brother-in-law's illness had a big impact on the whole family and none of us knew how to handle it. I approached the course in the way that I approached many things and that was to put my all into it. I pushed myself mentally.

I didn't experience the onset of my symptoms in the way that some people do, within a few hours or days after over exerting myself. My reaction to over-exertion was felt sometime after the event, by which time it was too late to stop a relapse. For this reason I learned to notice how I was feeling at regular intervals,

213

to monitor my feelings and any tension or aches in my body, so that I could stop and rest, or slow down, before I pushed myself too far.

I started to understand why I pushed myself continuously, to think how I set my objectives and goals in life and what value I put on things. It was great to see that I could look at things in a different way. I learned not to ignore any symptoms as I noticed them and to realise that I needed to change my point of view about a task or goal, before I suffered the consequences of pushing too hard.

An example of when I set myself a goal that was unrealistic was when I felt I had overeaten over a few days and wanted to lose some weight. I decided to walk to a certain location, regardless of how I was feeling and despite not having built myself up to walking that distance. My focus was on achieving my target, rather than on enjoying the activity and appreciating the experience of being outside in a beautiful park setting. I knew at the time that I was pushing myself too hard, but it wasn't until I talked about it that I realised how much more beneficial it would have been for me to set myself a more realistic target – to appreciate the view and being outdoors, rather than walking a certain distance because that is what I had set myself the target of doing. I have realised that being compassionate to myself is vital. In order to be well, I need to set myself realistic targets and enjoy what I am doing. The quality of an experience is much more important to me now.

Something I have learned, which has helped me recover from a relapse more quickly, is a relaxation technique which works for me. This, combined with being mindful and aware of how I am feeling, enables me to monitor my fatigue and take appropriate rests before I push myself to a point when relapse is inevitable. I am conscious too that alcohol can have an effect on my symptoms and so I avoid drinking too much.

I am aware now that thinking I will be well when I can do all the things I previously did is not helpful in my recovery. This is because doing all those things I used to do, and approaching them in the way I used to, contributed to me being ill. So now I know that accepting things will be different and that I can still lead a fulfilling enjoyable life is something important I have learned. My work with disabled people has demonstrated to me that it is possible to lead a life which is satisfying, and that it doesn't have to fit the pattern of so many people's extremely busy and hectic lives today. To believe that life will go back to the way it was before I had CFS/ME is something I have had to accept as being unrealistic. I know that it is my own ambitions and drive which are constant challenges to me. Prioritising my activities is important for managing how much I am doing. I also know it is important for me to incorporate something creative into my daily life, as well as remembering that doing pleasurable things in life is as important as achieving things.

I did keep a diary at times when I was suffering from a relapse and that helped me to look back and see what improvements I had made. It was a source of hope and encouragement to me to see that I was recovering. I think that keeping a diary when I am feeling well could help to identify more clearly the triggers for my relapses.

Chapter Eleven

Carers

Louise Penny and Sue Pemberton

Introduction

Caring for someone with a chronic illness such as CFS/ME brings its own demands and rewards. This chapter aims to offer an understanding of some of the consequences for people who have the condition and provide strategies for coping with chronic illness as a carer.

Are you a carer?

This is sometimes a term that we do not relate to ourselves, as we often consider that looking after someone is part and parcel of our relationship. This could be as a friend, relative, partner or child. You may have undertaken this role without hesitation when your loved one required further support, whether physical or emotional, and may not have initially recognised the impact that this has had upon all of your lives.

If you help someone who is ill, disabled or frail and that person depends upon you, you are a carer.

Caring is a broad term and can mean that you may just 'call in' on someone daily to check they are alright, or it may mean staying with that person 24 hours a day. No matter how small a role you feel you play, being a carer means devoting some of your time to somebody you care about, doing whatever you can to improve their quality of life.

What is chronic fatigue syndrome/ME?

Chronic fatigue syndrome/ME is a genuine and debilitating illness. Many people with the condition say that 'no-one can understand the condition who hasn't experienced it'. However, if anyone can come close to understanding the impact that it has, then it is the people who see how it affects someone every day.

It is not yet fully understood why people develop CFS/ME, and you may read about different medical views on the cause and treatment of the condition. This book is not intended to cover the varied theories around the triggers and processes of this health problem. However, from hearing the stories of so many people with CFS/ME, we have come to recognise some common patterns in the way in which the illness tends to develop. To help you to understand what someone may experience, we have compiled the common features into the most typical story of the illness.The following graphs help to explain a story of the development of CFS/ME, although we recognise that people can be different and not all of this may apply to the person you care for. In the next section we will explain this story looking at it one stage at a time.

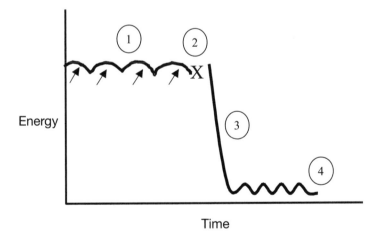

The energy pattern of CFS/ME

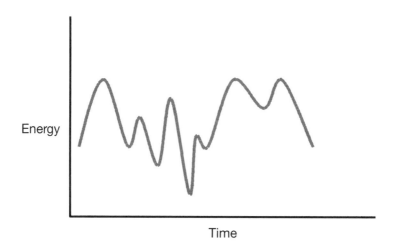

A normal energy pattern

The dotted line in the diagram above shows the normal fluctuating energy of someone who is healthy. It shows how our energy level changes all the time. Our bodies are designed to be 'switched on' (be active) and 'switch off' (relax). We all get 'tired', but usually our energy levels will pick up again.

Factors that may affect normal energy levels at any time would include:

- How much sleep we have had.
- Our diet and the amount of calories we have consumed.
- The internal demands on our body, such as fighting a virus or digesting food.
- How much energy we are using in different physical activities such as work, home or social activity.
- How much energy we are using in different mental or cognitive activities, such as prolonged periods of concentration or trying to solve problems.
- How much emotional energy is involved in our lives, such as stress at work, relationship difficulties or financial problems. Emotional energy

can also be positive and provide us with an 'energy boost'; imagine how you would feel if you won the lottery, passed your driving test or an exam?

- The time of day. Our natural body clock tells us when it is time to wind down and go to sleep, or wake up.

Energy patterns in CFS/ME

Different people who experience CFS/ME often describe a very similar story to their energy patterns before they became unwell. This story may also help you to understand why someone now is so different from how they were before.

1.   Some people describe how in the past they tended to push through the normal fluctuations of energy levels – trying to run on high energy more of the time in order to meet all the demands in their lives. Or they might just have been experiencing a busy time in their lives with lots going on, for example, when teenagers are preparing for exams.

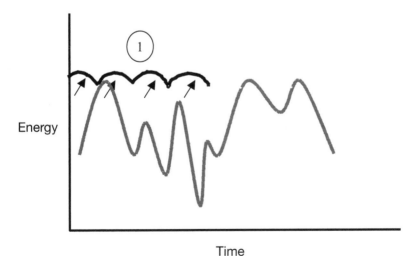

Some common features that people may use to describe themselves in the past are:

- Being a 'do-er' or leading a very active lifestyle.
- Feeling uncomfortable 'doing nothing' and finding it hard to relax.
- Being mentally very active, able to juggle plans for lots of different things in their heads at one time.
- Being very conscientious, not wanting to let people down. So, for example, they would push their energy levels to work late or by still meeting a commitment made to a friend when they felt unwell.
- Wanting to do things well – for example, wanting the house to look good or not wanting to make mistakes at work.
- Tending to put other's needs first, so using their energy to make sure other people were ok.
- Keeping going despite all. Maybe something happened in the person's life in the past, such as bereavement or financial pressures, which meant they had to keep going at that level to survive. This may also have meant that a lot of emotional energy was being utilised.

The first thing to notice is that this pattern does not have the normal 'switching on and off' and that the person is trying to run their body at the limits of their energy. As a carer, you may be able to relate to some of these features in the person you know, or in yourself.

2. Against this background, people with CFS/ME will often describe that there was some sort of 'trigger' to the condition. Although for some people it is more of a prolonged decline with a number of triggers.

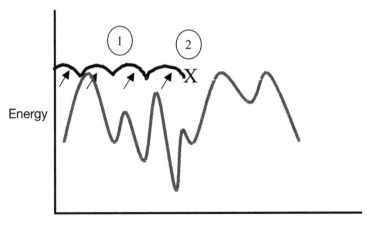

This could be a physical illness (such as a virus), a trauma (like an operation), a loss, a change in lifestyle or many other events. What seems to be common about all the triggers is that it is an extra demand on the body, which takes the person beyond what they can tolerate. Some people describe this as 'the straw that breaks the camel's back'.

This can make it difficult for carers to understand. As a carer you may have experienced the same trigger, such as having a cold or flu, or losing someone close, so why did you not get CFS/ME? It may be hard to understand why something seemingly simple to recover from, has caused such a disabling condition.

3. When people are first ill they start to experience a range of different and varying symptoms, such as fatigue, pain, headaches, sleep problems etc. Their energy level falls dramatically. But often people associate this with the trigger itself and do not think it is anything unusual. So, they may think 'I'll be better by next week' or 'When I get over this flu I'll be back at work'. They try to rest, maybe sleep more and try to recover.

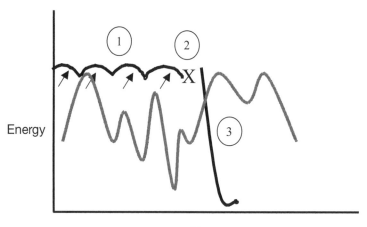

Time

4. What tends to occur in CFS/ME is that once the person's energy has
    picked up a little and they attempt to resume activity, they quickly find
    they cannot maintain it and their energy level falls again. Typically, the
    energy levels in CFS/ME fluctuate. The natural response appears to be
    that, when there is a little bit more energy, the person does more. This
    is often too much for the limited energy available and causes an increase
    in the symptoms. This is what we term 'boom and bust'.

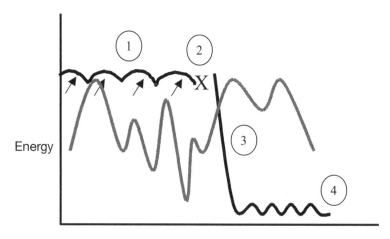

Time

The fluctuating nature of the fatigue, as well as being frustrating and confusing for the person themselves, adds to the difficulties for carers in understanding the condition and knowing what to do for the best. You may ask yourself, 'If they can do something one day, why can't they do it the next?' or 'Should I encourage them to do more or to rest more?'

In this book we have focused on enabling the person to establish a 'baseline' of activity. This means a level of activity that is sustainable (over good and bad days) which lessens the boom and bust cycle. Often the hardest part of this is to get people to hold back on the days when the energy seems to increase a little. There is no simple formula to finding a baseline, and it can take a long time for the individual to find the right level for themselves. Once a baseline is established, then they can gradually build up their activity levels at a pace that is achievable for them.

How can I help?

Carers play a vital role in supporting people to manage the condition. This can be in providing practical support for those jobs they cannot manage themselves, and providing emotional support to cope with the frustrations and distress that this condition can cause. People with CFS/ME are still able to laugh, but need someone to do this with. Therefore, there are lots of ways that you can help. Here are some suggestions:

- **Keep talking** - it is important to maintain open and honest communication, so discuss any worries or concerns you may have. People with CFS/ME still want to feel involved, but choose your moment. Discussion needs to take place when it is manageable to the person, such as when they are not too mentally or physically fatigued.

- **Be a good listener** – you cannot take away the symptoms but sometimes people just want someone to listen to them. They do not expect you to fix it. Feeling listened to and understood can go a long way towards relieving some of the frustration that goes with this condition.

- **Develop a greater understanding of the illness.** It is difficult to understand the condition as it keeps changing. These are some comments that people with the condition often report:
'When I had a little bit more energy and did more that day, everyone thought I was better.'
'Everyone thinks I look ok, so they don't understand how I feel inside.'
'My husband thinks I put my feet up all day, so why can't I have his dinner ready for him when he gets home.'

- **Be non-judgmental** – many people feel that they are thought to be lazy or unwilling, even when they are desperate to get better. Everyone experiences CFS/ME differently, so if you know others with the condition, do not always assume the same things will happen or work for them both.

- **Be encouraging** – focus on the things the person has achieved (however small) rather than how they were before the illness, or the things they cannot do.

- **Become involved** with their therapy; explore how you could help. You can read any information they may get from health professionals, ask about their therapy and see how you could help.

- **Help the person to maintain their baseline.** This may mean agreeing the tasks that you will do to help, and trying to remind them when they are doing too much. According to their ability, you may be able to support them in doing a little more over time.

- **Help the person to learn how to feel more relaxed.** Stress can have a big impact on fatigue levels, so wherever possible aim to reduce stress.

Maybe you could spend time doing something relaxing together, since it is also important for you to have relaxation time as well.

- **Encourage a partnership** between the person with the condition, members of the health team and yourself.

- **Look after yourself.** People with CFS/ME often feel guilty about the effect their illness is having on those around them. It is important that you still have time for yourself. Make sure that your needs are being met, and look after your own health.

How you may feel as a carer

We are all human and this condition will be affecting your life, as well as the life of the person who has it. It is common for carers, at times, to feel:

- Impatient with the person's behaviour.
- Angry and frustrated that doctors and others have not cured the problem.
- Worried that you are losing that person.
- Worried about coping and asking for help.
- Worried about the future, including financial concerns.
- Worried about the stigma associated with CFS/ME.
- Exhausted by listening and being the carer.
- Isolated from your usual social contacts.

Think about how you can get support as well. Do you have any friends or relatives who you can talk to, outside of the situation, to help you to keep going? There are also groups that may be able to help.

'Taking care of yourself' checklist

Make sure that you take time for yourself and do not ignore your own needs.

		Are you?
•	Sharing your worries with friends or family?	Yes / No
•	Asking for help if you are struggling? (We all have 'off days')	Yes / No
•	Making time for yourself to do leisure pursuits / catch up with your friends?	Yes / No
•	Remembering to exercise and eat healthily?	Yes/ No
•	Taking care of your own health concerns?	Yes / No
•	Asking for support from other family members or friends?	Yes / No
•	Asking to talk to a health or social care professional, if you need help?	Yes / No
•	Becoming involved in a carers' support group in your area?	Yes / No

---

Task

Write down what you could do to keep yourself healthy and what would support you in your caring role:

Sue's story

Jill is severely affected with CFS/ME and I have been her carer for eight years. At the beginning both Jill and I struggled to know what to do for the best, in terms of managing the illness that she is suffering from. She lives with me and at the start I did as much as I possibly could for her, including all of her personal care. I adjusted my speech, so that I talked in a quieter voice, because Jill was sensitive to noise. I also arranged for a bed to be moved into the living room for day time rests. We struggled with the emotional difficulties Jill was experiencing, and I was living with the illness just as much as Jill was.

In time, I began to separate the illness which Jill has from the person she is. It was difficult for Jill's CFS/ME not to become the focus of our lives. As I began to see past the CFS/ME and see Jill as a person with the condition, the quality of our lives improved. I used to read everything I could about CFS/ME. It is important to have an understanding of the illness, but not to let it take over.

Our lives were turned around after we came under the care of a specialist service. It was important for Jill to regain some independence and to build up her self-esteem. We were shown how to break down the task of putting on socks, for example, into tiny manageable steps. After two to three months, Jill achieved this goal. Thus began the slow and painful progress of her regaining some independence in her personal care.

Another key step was to accept the support of friends and neighbours who lived close by. One of them, Linda, spent time with Jill and has become one of her greatest friends. She is a great listener and she draws on her own personal experiences to encourage and support Jill. She can often see some of the things I struggle with more clearly, probably because I am so close to Jill and her illness. I have found it difficult to know how to support her at times. There have been oc-casions when Jill has had a good day and I have responded by saying that maybe the following day she could do even more. This has felt like pressure and even criticism to Jill. I have learned that sometimes, when she is feeling particularly ill and tearful, the best thing I can do is to agree that she is having a bad time and how difficult it must be to be so ill. In the past I would have tried to lift her out of her low mood, when sometimes she simply needs love and reassurance. I find I can empathise with her much more now. Communication is so important and being a good listener to Jill is often what she needs. Talking late in the day doesn't work for her and so if we have something to discuss we make sure that we do it when she is feeling well enough. Jill felt a lot of frustration and anger with her illness and I found that difficult, because it was directed at me as I was the one she was spending her time with. I also found it difficult because I have not experienced those emotions myself. I tried to see past the emotions and understand that it wasn't personal to me. Having the support of friends and specialist professionals has helped Jill and me to see things from a different point of view at times and to understand each other better.

Constant adjusting and adapting is needed, because on some days Jill can do more than on others. Her energy fluctuates and on some days she will decide not to get dressed because she wants to use her energy for something else. Getting the right balance of when to help and when to stand back is difficult. Jill may tell me, or write a list of, what she hopes to achieve, for example, as part of preparing lunch. They will be very small, achievable steps, over a period of time. This means Jill is making decisions and asking for what she needs help with and her self-confidence is growing.

I have always been included in Jill's treatment and I think it is important to work as a team, with each other and with the medical professionals who support her. I've learned the importance of having time for myself, and I have my interests and breaks.

Jill has developed a sense of humour about herself and that has helped us both enormously. We can now laugh about some of the difficulties she faces and she doesn't take things as personally as she previously did. We are able to enjoy life. Pleasure is important. Jill's illness has been a physical, mental and emotional rollercoaster for us both. With her hard work and all the support we get, we are positive about the future. She has a quality of life. We are getting back to normal – whatever that is!

Index

adrenaline and 96
body's response to demand/threat 95-7
    survival and 95-7
case study: Jill 110-13
definition of 93-5
diet and *see* Diet
demands on energy, 94-7
distraction 106-8
fatigue and 100
flight or fight response 96
lifestyle and 109
management of 100-1
relaxation 101-13
    see also Relaxation
response to stress, assessment of 98-100
signs of 99-100
    behavioural 100, 101
    emotional 99, 100, 101
    irritable bowel system (IBS) 103
    physical 99, 101, 102
sleep and *see* Sleep
thoughts, awareness of 106
Stress response
    biological pathway 97-8
    parasympathetic nervous system 97-8,
        100, 101
    sympathetic nervous system 97-8
Supplements 74

Tasks for
    activity and energy 9, 19, 27, 33, 37
    memory 152, 156, 160-1
    relapse 208
    sleep 61-2
    stress 99-100, 101, 105, 107-8
    thoughts 120-1, 125
Thinking errors 132
Thinking patterns 132-3
Thoughts and feelings 114-49
    anger 121, 124, 128
    anxiety 116,120, 121, 123, 124, 128, 147

    see also Anxiety
    assumptions 118-9
    automatic thoughts 118-9, 136-8, 138
    behaviour and 118-9
    biases in thinking 121-2
    case study: David, 147-9
    challenging your thoughts 130-42, 148
        alternative thoughts, development of
            136-8
        evidence for and against each
            thought 134-8
        examples 131, 141, 140
        techniques for 134-8
    change and loss, dealing with 116
    cognitive behavioural therapy (CBT)
        117-27
    cognitive biases 132
    connections
        between thoughts and behaviour
            125-6
        between thoughts and emotions
            122-3
        between thoughts and feelings 121-3
        between thoughts and physical
            reactions 123-4
        between thoughts and present
            situation 119-21
    core beliefs 118-9
    demoralisation, 114
    depression 116, 121, 123
    definition of 142-3
        see also Depression
    diary, thought 127-30, 132-3
    distortions, of thoughts 132
    emotions and mood 118-19
    frustration 114, 128
    guilt 117, 121, 123
    levels of thought 117-19
    management of 117-18
    mood, low 16
        management of 142-3
    negative thoughts, monitoring of
        127-30

What You Need to Know About
Pernicious Anaemia & Vitamin B12 Deficiency

Martyn Hooper MBE

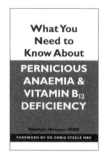

Vitamin B12 deficiency arising from dietary, digestive or autoimmune issues can be a significant cause of unremitting fatigue. Martyn Hooper MBE, founder of the Pernicious Anaemia Society, draws on the experience of the Society's 7000+ members to explain why diagnosis is so often missed and why problems continue for many sufferers even after diagnosis and treatment.

'This book will be essential reading for all who suffer from pernicious anaemia and for those who suspect that they might be deficient in vitamin B12. It is very clearly written in a style that is both entertaining and instructive. Although written for a lay audience, it is soundly based on good science and could be read with profit by physicians, who need to be made more aware of this health problem.'
David Smith, Professor Emeritus of Pharmacology,
University of Oxford, UK